'Payal—whatever I say about her will never be enough! Her smile and absolutely loving nature got to me instantly. When I did my first yoga class with her and saw her in a yogic posture, I just knew I had found my yoga tutor for life. Her dedication to my body, her perseverance, loyalty, and commitment have helped me challenge my genes and transform my body to what it is today—from not being able to do five Suryanamaskars to doing 108 in the first five months is what Payal took me to. She has such a natural flair for yoga that even when she makes me do the toughest asana it becomes so easy! Her calming nature and the understanding she has shown towards my body is something I can never forget. Thank you Payal, thank you for yelling at me in every class but always with your loving smile. To me yoga is not a part of my life; it is my way of living and always will be!'

Kareena Kapoor

'To be an excellent instructor you must be able to inspire and motivate your client. You must know how to push them and encourage them to willingly cross their limits of endurance. Payal does all this and more. I find her classes to be very challenging and look forward to them.'

Saif Ali Khan

'I feel like Payal has been not just a teacher, but someone who has been part of a journey with me. She is the instrument of change that helped me discover a more holistic approach to life. She is a very good trainer and has helped me do my best every single day.'

Rani Mukerji

'Payal's yoga is the best thing to have happened to me. It's been sometime since I have been practising this form of yoga and it has done wonders to my lifestyle and me. The entire process of learning yoga from Payal and her husband Manish has been very rewarding for me. Her form of yoga neither strains nor exhausts your body and mind. Apart from being physically fit and agile, my mind is completely at peace. I have been so satisfied that I have even introduced my children to yoga.'

Sridevi Kapoor

'Payal is a wonderfully positive person who makes the experience of yoga and exercise so delightful. It was enlighten-ment to find a teacher like her.'

Jacqueline Fernandez

'Payal has been super. Yoga and Payal have changed my life!'
Amrita Arora Ladak

'I love working with Payal. She is a person who pushes you for sure but in a nice way, and to work out and sustain your workouts you need a gentle push. Her exercises make me feel great and more energetic as it is a beautiful blend of spiritualism and exercise.'

Priya Dutt

'Payal introduced me to the world of yoga and thereby made a huge difference to my level of fitness. She is very knowledgeable and sincere at the same time. On my first day, I found the postures very tough. However, thanks to her enthusiasm, I began enjoying the pain and the struggle that comes with being a beginner. Today I can't think of leaving and the credit for it goes to Payal.'

Tusshar Kapoor

'I love working out with Payal because each workout seems absolutely different. I'm never completely tired after Payal's workout instead I'm completely charged for a brand new day. She is fun, encouraging and pushes you to *your* limits, not *hers*, and that is I think the deciding factor between a good yoga teacher and an excellent one. As for me, I'm always game to go back for more.'

Maria Goretti

'Payal is a dedicated and a reliable professional who is not only very passionate about what she does but also delivers results.'

Tulip Joshi

'Payal's Suryanamaskars are like magic. When I'm out of the country and have no time to train, I do 50 Suryanamaskars in the morning. It takes me just 20 minutes and I am able to maintain the bikini body through the holiday. It also helps to digest food faster and keeps my body free of toxins. Thank you Payal for showing me how to come back guilt free from my holidays!'

Zoa Morani

'Experience Payal's yoga techniques and you will thank me always.'

Malaika Arora Khan

from
XL
to XS

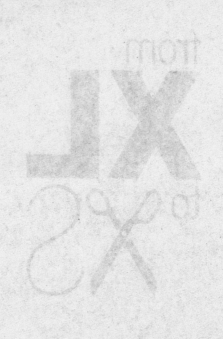

from
XL
to XS

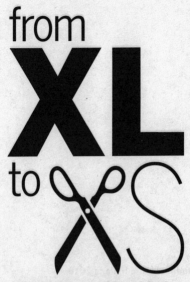

A fitness guru's guide to
changing your body

Payal Gidwani Tiwari

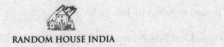

RANDOM HOUSE INDIA

Published by Random House India in 2010
3

Copyright © Payal Gidwani Tiwari 2010
Black & white yoga photographs by Ryan Martis

Random House Publishers India Private Limited
MindMill Corporate Tower, 2nd Floor, Plot No 24A
Sector 16A, Noida 201301, UP

Random House Group Limited
20 Vauxhall Bridge Road
London SW1V 2SA, UK

978-81-8400-147-1

This book is sold subject to the condition that it shall not, by way of trade
or otherwise, be lent, resold, hired out, or otherwise circulated without the
publisher's prior consent in any form of binding or cover other than that in
which it is published and without a similar condition including this condition being imposed on the subsequent purchaser.

Typeset in Sabon by Jojy Philip

Printed and bound in India by Replika Press.

To my parents

Contents

Acknowledgements

Before I can even collect my thoughts, I would like to thank the almighty, the supreme power, for making me the medium to reach out to the world in my own little way through this book.

My celebrity clients who not only took out their valuable time to share their thoughts, tips, and experiences and shoot pictures for the book, but also allowed me to share their exercise routines with their fans.

My teacher Suchint Kaur Sodhi, senior yoga guru, Kaivailyadhyam Lonavala, who helped me with her valuable inputs for the book.

My students, for bearing with my irregular presence and for their wholehearted support throughout the writing of this book.

My cousin Ekta Mohanani Kamra who generously volunteered to model for the yoga pictures in the book.

My best friend and HR manager Hemali Punjabi, and the teachers and staff at my studio Cosmic Fusion, who looked after it beautifully while I took time off to write.

My in-laws for their encouragement and understanding even though I could not spend enough time with them on their annual visit.

My brother Sahil, my bhabhi Meet, mummy (my grand-mother), daddy (my late grandfather), and all of my extended family—my buas, uncles, cousins—who have always stood by me in all my ventures including this one.

Chotu, my cook, who kept us all well-fed during the writing of the book; Imran and Rajesh, my drivers, who were always there when I needed them.

Milee Ashwarya, my editor, without whom this book could never have got the structure and form it has now.

And lastly, my loving hubby Manish, the most important person in my life, without whom this book and my life would have been incomplete.

Introduction

If I were to ask you, which were the happiest days of your life, most of you would reply, your school days. Have you ever wondered why? Why do we always cherish our childhood? Is it because back then, we had no real responsibilities or that life wasn't so competitive? No, not exactly. Even in school we had things to worry about, like getting good grades in exams, taking part in sports, and preparing for extracurricular activities. Didn't we have to face peer pressure, comparison with siblings, bullying by seniors, and problems at home among other things? So what was the difference? The answer is simple. It's because of the time that we spent playing and running about.

As we grow, we take on more and more work and responsibilities but start ignoring our bodies. We have a million things to worry about; be it related to our career, love life, family, society, money, status, etc. Along the way we often forget to take out time to play or physically exert ourselves in any way. And I believe this is the cause of most of our health-related problems today.

When I was in school, I was nicknamed 'rubber band' as I could twist and turn my body in any possible way. This of course came in very handy later when I took up yoga. But coming back to school, academics was never my forte. What I loved, however, was sports, especially athletics—long jump, high jump, short put, or javelin. Never a bookworm, I thrived on outdoor activities. I still remember getting into my shorts and running up and down the slope around my parents' Bandstand residence in Bandra, Mumbai, during my summer break. I used to consistently get an A+ in sports and so when I was made the physical-education prefect of my school, no one was surprised.

When I graduated from school, physical training was not yet a very popular or sought after career choice. Fitness experts were unheard of, and were at best few and far in between. So I studied interior design, which was considered a safer profession. I did quite a few projects, but deep down I was not totally happy. I felt like I was missing something, and that's when I thought I should get back to doing what I enjoyed the most and turn my gift into my profession. But I was not sure how to go about it; which road to take to make the best use of my gift. Eventually, in 2003, I opted for yoga as it is a holistic way to good health. I told myself that I would try it out for six months and see whether it worked for me or not. As fate would have it, I was hooked. That's how I started my journey as a physical trainer. It has been seven years since and I've never looked back.

Fitness to me is a combination of many things—a good body, flexibility, endurance, strength, good skin and hair, restful sleep—and you can achieve all this with the help of yoga. Many people ask me how yoga differs from other forms of exercise, and why they should follow this ancient form of exercise when there are so many new and exciting options around.

First, yoga works on your internal organs. The exercises massage the internal organs. For instance, when you do Paschimottanasana and bend forward, your hamstring is stretched, your hip area opens up completely, and your internal organs like the spleen, stomach, and intestines are kneaded, due to which there is an extra flow of blood to the nerves and muscles. This helps in their better functioning, and makes you healthy inside out.

Second, yoga teaches you the right way to breathe and to control your breathing. It connects with basic and fundamental aspects of daily life. Did you know that just by breathing properly you could control ageing? Third, yoga propels you on the path of self-realization. With regular practice, you can understand yourself better, and learn to control your anger as well as various negativities and urges. Fourth, there is a popular myth that 'yoga doesn't make you lose weight'. This is absolutely incorrect. I can safely vouch for yoga as a means of losing weight, as this is what I have been doing over the years, helping people lose weight and making them look more beautiful. If done in the right way, yoga can definitely help you lose weight and that too naturally, without popping pills and taking fat burners. And all this without any side effects. When you hold an asana for more than a minute, it melts the fat cells and helps you to reduce weight. For instance, Utkatasana or the 'chair pose' melts fat from the thigh area, the butt, and the calves. You can lose kilos or inches with diets as well, but you can never look toned. You have to exercise to prevent your body from looking flabby and shrivelled.

Fifth, yoga consists of certain inverted postures or asanas in which you have to bend down and the blood flows to the head and other areas. Such inverted postures are unique only to yoga and do not form a part of any other form of exercise. When the blood flow is directed towards these organs, it lends an extra glow to the face and the skin. Such exercises can even cure ailments like migraine, sinusitis, asthma, acne, etc., and turn grey hair black again. I will talk about it in more detail in the chapter related to ageing.

Lastly, and most importantly, yoga can change the shape of your body. Often I come across people who are slim, yet not satisfied with their bodies. They have different problem areas that they constantly worry about, like for example, their hands might be too thin, they might have a hint of a double chin or they feel that their waist is a little broader than what they prefer. However, through regular practice of yoga you can get the body you dream of and look at yourself in the mirror with confidence and pride. By working on your specific problem areas, you can change the structure of your body. And by following your workout regularly, you can become a perfect ten with a perfectly proportionate body.

So with yoga, I make beautiful people look more beautiful. And this brings me to my connection with Bollywood. It all happened to me by chance when one day I got a call from Bebo. Yes, she was my first celebrity client. Celebrities come with higher expectations, and have set goals with deadlines in mind, but in my experience, they are also the most dedicated and hardworking people that I have ever worked with. It is challenging in a way as well, because you have to make sure that you deliver within the time frame. And this forces you to be extremely disciplined, think out of the box, focus better, and adjust the regime to the individual in order to meet the desired goal. Working with them has helped me make my workouts better and more effective. Their focus and commitment towards their bodies is outstanding.

Where did I get the inspiration for the book? Last year I accompanied Bebo and Saif to New York for the shooting of *Kurbaan*. We had a great time in New York and even managed to add to their exercise routine by doing two yoga classes in Central Park. It felt so refreshing to be practising yoga in the ideal natural surroundings. As we sat in the Mumbai airport international lounge, Saif looked up to me and said, 'Payal, you must share what you do with everybody.' It was unlike Saif and I was too surprised to say anything at that time, but it did get me thinking. And when I was approached by Random House to write a book, I decided to take on the opportunity to reach out to many more people all across the country who want to look good but don't know how to do it.

Losing weight and looking beautiful is all in your hands. And believe me it is not so difficult. It is more like a habit that you have to adopt in your normal lifestyle. And you don't need much, just about an hour a day, to stay healthy, young, and beautiful. Surely, you can take one hour out for yourself. We all can.

Mumbai
September 2010

How to use this book

Losing weight might take a while but it is possible and I feel anybody can do it. Chapter 1 is about finding out how many kilos overweight you are by, and then setting about losing them. I have specific workouts in the book for people with different kinds and categories of weight issues, and you can lose weight by following them diligently.

After you have reached your ideal body weight, you can work towards changing the shape of your body. I have exercise routines based on different body shapes in Chapter 2, so you can work on your weak areas, and achieve a perfect ten figure.

The third chapter is for people who want to go a step further and improve their level of fitness. So here I talk about how to improve your flexibility, endurance, and strength, which are key factors for overall fitness. I have included a brief Chapter 4 at the end of Part One, which tells you how to use the various workouts in this book according to your specific needs. I have detailed how you can incorporate a specific regime in your workout in case you have already been working out.

In the second part of the book, I talk about the invisible factors of good health which significantly affect the way we look. Ageing is a reality that all of us have to deal with sooner or later. In Chapter 5, I talk about how you can look ten years younger than your real age. Yes, it is possible! I also share some beauty tips and regimes of stars, and offer tips to deal with aches and pains.

Beauty is something we all bother about and covet. Did you know that there are specific exercises for our skin, hair, and eyes? In chapter six, the Bollywood beauties and I will share with you the secret of looking more beautiful. The last chapter of the book delves into some other important factors of looking fresh and attractive, like getting a good night's sleep and dealing with stress. These are day-to-day things that we ignore but they nonetheless, play an important role in how we look.

At the back of the book, I have included a crash course in yoga for people who do not have any specific goal in mind, but nevertheless want to stay healthy and fit. I have categorized the course into three levels—beginners, elementary, and advanced—depending upon what stage you are in. And lastly, I have also included a chronological list of all exercises mentioned in the book with explanations and their benefits detailed so that when you are doing a particular exercise, you know how to do it and also what it does to your body. I suggest you read the directions carefully before attempting any exercise.

From XL to XS is a practical and result-oriented book and what I have shared here with you is what has successfully worked for many people whom I have worked with. I have always believed in natural remedies like yoga as it is the only long lasting and reliable solution to the problems of this new millennium. There are many shortcuts and quick fixes available in the market but those will only ruin your health in the long run. So it is best to make the right choice today than regret tomorrow when it is too late.

About the exercises

The contents of this book are based on my personal and professional experiences. Yoga does not require complicated techniques, so you can easily follow the routines in the book, if you have already been doing yoga. Also, due care has been taken to make sure that there are photographs, directions, and precautions for most exercises in the book. However, in case you are new to yoga, it is advisable to practise it under the supervision of a yoga expert, so that you do not get injured. The author or the publisher will not bear any responsibility for any aches and pains, injuries, or discomfort caused by doing the exercises in this book.

Part One

In the Eyes

1

How to lose or gain weight

I was seventeen when I met Payal for the first time. Even then I knew I wanted to become an actress but I was fat and underconfident. I would look at other slim and fit girls and wish I could be like them. And then my life changed. I was fifty-three kilos when I started working out with Payal in 2005. Within a year I had lost seven kilos and come down to forty-six kilos. Not only that, I had lost around 40 inches in that one year. My body started shaping up, my eating habits changed, and I became more focused towards everything in my life.

You know how it is when you look and feel good about yourself. My friends and family certainly noticed it and were, in fact, surprised to see me in my new avatar. As for me, I was happy, and so were my parents seeing my positive attitude towards life. And the credit for all this goes to Payal. She has worked really hard to help me lose weight and get in shape. I was young and restless but Payal kept on motivating me. She was like a strict yet loving second mom, always there for me especially when my mom was out of town. She would make sure that I remained focused and did my workouts on time. In fact, she would scold me if I didn't do my exercises. But I think all that has made me what I am today.

I strongly believe that yoga is a blessing and anybody who has done it would know what I am talking about. It changes your life, not just your body, and your mind. My childhood dream is finally coming true and Payal has a huge hand in it since it was she who made me look and feel like an actress. Honestly, I do think that if I can, then anybody can lose weight and step into that little black dress with confidence!

Zoa Morani

Are you overweight?

Most of us struggle with weight issues today. With the kind of lifestyle we lead and the food culture we are growing up with, it is very easy to put on weight. We are increasingly getting addicted to electronic gadgets and it is common to spend hours watching TV, working or playing games on the computer, tweeting friends, checking and updating our facebook or orkut profiles, texting on the phone, and so on. While a few decades back we would spend our evenings doing things like playing a sport, meeting friends, walking in the park, now we increasingly stay indoors. There is home delivery for everything so why waste time going out and getting something when you get everything at the mere touch of your fingertips? Moreover, we love to play around with these gadgets and sometimes even end up getting addicted to them. And doesn't it make sense to keep up with the fad? What will our friends think otherwise?

All these habits make us lazy and sedentary, and as a result we put on weight. Then there is a growing trend of junk, fried, readymade, or instant food. Chips (and there are hundred varieties to choose from), noodles, pastas, colas, doughnuts, patties are the instant answer to our hunger pangs. But what we do not realize is that these are fattening and difficult to digest.

When Priya Grover, a 34-year-old working woman, came to me she weighed seventy-five kilos. Her ideal weight, as per her height of 5 feet 7 inches, was sixty-one to sixty-five kilos, so she was roughly ten kilos overweight. And to make matters worse, she was putting on more weight with each passing month. Priya had a sweet tooth and she loved desserts; chocolates, brownies, ice creams, pastries, gulab jamuns, you name it. Although she was trying to control her weight, instead of going down, it was spiralling upwards. She had also started experiencing sharp mood swings and would get irritated at trivial things.

I have often noticed that the late twenties to mid-thirties is a very crucial phase for women. This is the time when our bodies change significantly and it is very easy to put on weight. As we age, the metabolic rate of our bodies slows down and we do not burn up calories as easily as we used to do before, when we were in school or college. There are also certain hormonal changes taking place in the body that make it easier to put on weight and more difficult to lose it as we age.

Another common reason is that in India this is the time when most women get married and then start ignoring their bodies. Some get pregnant very soon, and have to deal with the weight gain during pregnancy. Isn't this phenomenon common? Most Indian couples put on weight soon after they get married. They get so busy adjusting to their new lifestyle, home, and families that they don't realize when and how their bodies change. Yes, it is true. Even girls who have been really thin in their teenage years start putting on weight. I feel that the first six months after your wedding are really crucial as this is the time when you can either be careless and pile on kilos or be conscious of your weight and save yourself a lot of worry later on. I feel this is the phase when you need to make an extra effort to stay fit. Putting on weight is easy, but it gets more and more difficult to lose it. I am glad that Priya came to me while she was overweight and before she had turned obese. Even then, it took her a full year to shed all the extra kilos. But at 35 she was slim and smiling, and looked much younger than she used to when I had first seen her.

Am I overweight or am I obese?

Being overweight is really common nowadays. I meet people from all walks of life who are overweight if not obese. But what is obesity and when are you overweight? And how are the two different? When you consume more calories than you can use or burn out, you start accumulating the excess calories in your body as fat. This gets deposited as a layer under your skin. You are overweight when you cross the threshold of your ideal body weight.

So, for example, if you are 5 feet 2 inches and your ideal body weight is fifty-four kilos but you are sixty-two kilos, then you are overweight. However, if your weight is 30 per cent more than your ideal body weight you will be termed obese.

Obesity is literally, an advanced stage of being overweight, and actually a disease which can lead to serious medical conditions like high blood pressure and other heart diseases, diabetes, osteoporosis, digestive problems, sleep disorders, backache, and many more.

Body Mass Index or BMI is used to ascertain whether you are overweight or not, and by how much. It is calculated on the basis of your weight and your height.

$$BMI= W/H^2$$

For example, if you are 5 feet 3 inches and weigh fifty-two kilos, your BMI will approximately be 20. What I have done here is converted your height into metres; so in this case it is 1.6 metres, and then divided it by your weight, which is the number of kilos by the square of your height.

So we have,

$$52/1.6 \times 1.6 = 20.3$$

If your BMI is less than 18, then you are underweight. However, if your BMI is between 18 to 25, you are considered to be normal. In case your BMI is 25 or more, then you are overweight. Here, too, there are different categories; so if your BMI is between 25–30 then you are overweight but still in the pre-obesity stage. However, if your BMI is more than 30, it indicates obesity, and you seriously need to do something about it.

Interestingly, fat or adipose tissues are formed in most of us right in our childhood. And once these tissues are formed they keep troubling us intermittently. Don't we all adore plump babies? But what most of us don't realize is that we are harming them by over feeding them and making them lethargic and dull. This is really a troubling trend. In fact, I have noticed a sudden rise in obesity among children in the past five years or so. Most of these cases are a result of the parents' negligence as infants eat only what is given to them.

Although there are many reasons for putting on weight, the most common ones are wrong eating habits, overeating, and leading a sedentary lifestyle, or even a combination of all these factors. You might not be getting enough time to exercise due to a heavy workload, which leaves you feeling exhausted by the end of the day. I have also met many people who have a complete lack of motivation to lose weight, and do not take fitness seriously. Some of them feel that since they are not in the spotlight or don't have to face the camera, it doesn't matter much. However, the most common category is of people who love to eat and are not very disciplined with their diet or exercise. Such people don't mind putting on a couple of extra kilos as they think it is no big deal, and wouldn't really make them look out of shape. This reminds me of my client Michelle Thomas, an effervescent banker who puts on around five to seven kilos every year during Christmas and New Year, and spends the rest of the year burning it out.

When you are overweight, you have the opportunity of losing weight sooner than when you crossover into the obese category. In fact, in some cases you can immediately get back to your ideal body weight by just making a few alterations in your daily routine like correcting your diet, doing a 30-minute physical routine and getting out of your sedentary lifestyle.

However, when you are obese, it takes substantially more time, effort, dedication, and discipline to get back into shape.

Before we get started

Step one: Motivation is in your pocket

Often I have heard my clients say, 'I know I am fat, and I need to lose weight. But I am so busy; I just don't have the time to exercise.'

The hard truth is that these are just excuses. Motivation is near you—with you—but you just can't see it. It is in your pocket, you just have find it. Just like we make time for eating, sleeping, and other things that we consider important, the same way we can find the time for exercising. Taking care of your body is as important, if not more, than other things in your life. So the next time you say you don't have time for exercising, remember that you are just making excuses or being plain lazy.

There are also some others who just don't want to think about losing weight. They feel that they are too fat or too old to lose weight. Or worse, have crossed the threshold from where there is no way back. They hate to look at themselves in the mirror and avoid even going near the weighing scales. In short, they have totally given up hope. So don't these people actually want to lose weight? Of course they do! They just don't think it is possible anymore. I want to tell all of them that 'you can'.

When Divya Thavani came to me, my first reaction was: what a beautiful girl! She was a 20-year-old student, tall, (around 5 feet 8 inches) and extremely attractive. But Divya weighed hundred and twenty kilos! And she didn't know what to do about it. She felt that she was so fat, that there was no hope left for her. Divya's problem was a combination of hereditary obesity, careless eating habits, and lack of exercise. She would have some form of junk food almost every day. But after I started working with Divya, believe me, she became one of my most dedicated students. She has already lost ten kilos in just forty-five days and I'm sure that within a year, she will be able to come down to her ideal body weight of sixty-two to sixty-seven kilos.

You too can lose weight and embrace good health. You too can wear whatever you want, and look young and beautiful. Why wear loose clothes to hide your waist or your belly? Why wear maternity clothes when you are not pregnant?

You just need to take out a minimum of around 30 minutes to a maximum of 90 minutes for yourself to exercise, and I strongly believe that you owe that to yourself and your body. There is no age or stage in life to start taking care of your body. The day you wake up is the day your new life begins. Good health is for everybody. Make a fresh start today.

Step two: Know your ideal body weight

Body weight is something that bothers each one of us today and will continue to do so in the times to come. Ironically, the lifeless weighing scale is our worst enemy. Those who are trying to lose weight hate it and so do the ones who are trying to gain weight as the figures on the weighing scale are never satisfactory. So what is this ideal body weight that all of us are searching for?

Ideal body weight is one of the most important markers

Tips for getting motivated

- Look at yourself in a full-length mirror without any clothes. The mirror will show you the truth; exactly what your body looks like and where you need to lose weight.
- Buy a weighing machine and keep it in your bedroom. Check your weight regularly, and it'll help you keep a tab on your weight.
- Look at your old pictures, maybe of your school or college days when you were thinner.
- Try out your old clothes, and see if you fit into those or not.
- Keep in touch with your old friends. They will tell you how you looked before.
- Don't be a step behind; match steps with your children. Become your daughter's or son's partner while working out.
- Set a specific goal for yourself. It can be anything like—I have to fit into that black dress, or I want to shed seven kilos before my anniversary, etc.
- Get your friends or neighbours together and workout with them while chatting, watching your favourite TV soaps, etc.

of fitness. It is nothing but what your weight should be as per your height, age, gender, and body structure. So, needless to say, it is different for different people. Every bone structure can carry only a particular amount of kilos comfortably. Any excess weight will apply stress on the joints, back, etc., and attract other health problems like high cholesterol, heart blockage, diabetes, etc. A balance between the weight and the height of a particular body structure is a must and can be achieved through a healthy diet, physical training, and mental balance. I believe it is very important to know your ideal body weight before going on any kind of diet or exercise regime. Getting to know your ideal body weight is the first step towards fitness. Once you know your ideal body weight, you can figure out how many kilos overweight you are and how many kilos you need to lose.

The next step would be to find out how much time you need to lose the extra kilos that you have piled on, and then start working towards losing them earnestly. What I find surprising is that most of the people who workout, do not know what

Stretch marks

How do we develop stretch marks? When the skin expands over its capacity and shrinks suddenly, you end up having stretch marks on your body. These are most commonly seen in obese people, women post pregnancy, body builders, or even in adolescents during puberty. Abdomen, breasts, upper arms, back, thighs, buttocks, etc., are the areas most prone to stretch marks.

What can you do to prevent stretch marks? Moisturize your entire body regularly with cocoa butter or a vitamin-E-based lotion. In case of a sudden change in your body weight, start applying it religiously. Don't wait for the marks to appear! Be proactive and apply it on your entire body regularly as soon as your weight starts fluctuating. And remember, stretch marks go away only with time. So don't expect instant results, as you will only be disappointed.

their ideal body weight is. They keep on exercising blindly, and just worry about the inches or the kilos that they have shed. But this is a wrong approach. What might be the ideal body weight for someone else with the same age and height might not be the ideal weight for you. That is the reason, in Table 1.1, we have a range for the ideal body weight even for people with the same height and weight.

We all have different body types. Some of us are small framed while some others are medium or large. You must have heard someone saying, 'I have really heavy bones.' Bone weight or bone density also contributes to the overall weight of your body. The fat percentage in each person is also different as each of us is unique with our own strengths and weaknesses. No wonder then that the ideal body weight of a Western woman would be different from that of an Indian woman of the same height, and even among Indian women of the same height it would differ. However, you can find out your ideal body weight if you like with the help of an expert.

We live in a tech savvy world and with TV, films, and internet reigning in our lives, we are aware of all that is happening in the rest of the world. Unconsciously or consciously, we try to ape the West, and in this case the Hollywood actresses and models, who are extremely thin, bony, and tall. We run after fashion rather than fitness. But what we tend to forget is that they have a different body type and structure, and we Indians have totally different bodies. Indian women have curvaceous bodies with heavier chests and hips, especially the women from north and south India. So the bottom line is: no matter how much you try, you cannot look like Western women. And the truth is that Indian men like voluptuous women. So don't think that you need to look like a European model to please your man!

Unless you know what your body needs, how can you give that to it? Just as without the right goal in mind, can you even think of achieving it? So first you need to know your body well. Remember, if you do things right the first time, you won't have to do them again. Look at the table on the next page, which will give you an approximate idea of the ideal body weight for you, and consequently the number of kilos that you need to lose. This is a goal that you can set up for yourself, and it's always better to work towards a specific goal.

Table 1.1 will help you find out your ideal body weight. There is a separate column to show if you are overweight or not. If you are more than the maximum number of kilos mentioned in the overweight table, then you will fall into the pre-obesity and obesity categories.

Table 1.1 Ideal body weight

Height (Feet & metres)	Ideal Weight for Men (kilos)	Ideal Weight for Women (kilos)	Overweight if in the range for Men in (kilos)	Overweight if in the range for Women (kilos)
5'-0" (1.523 m)	51–54	51–54	54–59.4	54–59.4
5'-1" (1.548 m)	52–55	52–55	55–60.5	55–60.5
5'-2" (1.574 m)	56–60	53–57	60–66	57–62.7
5'-3" (1.599 m)	58–62	54–58	62–68.2	58–63.8
5'-4" (1.624 m)	59–63	56–60	63–69.3	60–66
5'-5" (1.650 m)	61–65	58–61	65–71.5	61–67.1
5'-6" (1.675 m)	62–67	59–62	67–73.7	62–68.2
5'-7" (1.700 m)	64–68	61–65	68–74.8	65–71.5
5'-8" (1.726 m)	66–71	62–67	71–78.1	67–73.7
5'-9" (1.751 m)	68–72	64–68	72–79.2	68–74.8
5'-10" (1.777 m)	69–75	66–70	74–82.5	70–77
5'-11" (1.802 m)	71–76	67–72	76–83.6	72–79.2
6'-0" (1.827 m)	73–79	68–74	79–86.9	74–81.4
6'-1" (1.853 m)	73–81	73–81	81–89.1	81–89.1
6'-2" (1.878 m)	77–84	78–83	84–92.4	83–91.3
6'-3" (1.904 m)	80–86	80–85	86–94.6	85–93.5

Step three: Deal with water retention

What most of us don't know is that it is not always fat that contributes to weight gain. Many a times, it is fluids that add to your body weight. In fact, water retention is one of the main causes of weight gain. I come across so many women who keep on complaining, 'Even though I eat healthy and exercise regularly, I'm not able to lose weight. I feel *so* frustrated'.

This is because their weight is not only the result of fat deposition but also water accumulation in the muscles and the cavities of the body. So if you want to lose weight normally and get quick results like others you must find out whether you have water retention in your body or not.

I have a simple test to find out if a person has water retention or not. Press the skin on your thigh or your arms and if the skin wrinkles after you pinch it, you have water retention. You can do it yourself and see if you have water retention in your body or not.

The next step is to get this excess water out of your system. How can you do it? Most people would start drinking even lesser amounts of water, not realizing that water deficiency is what leads to water retention. So the less water you drink, the more water will get accumulated in your body. What happens is that when we drink less than the required amount of water, our kidneys cannot filter out all the toxins from the body. These toxins or fluids then get stored in the muscles, making them weak and flabby. The most susceptible areas for water retention are all big muscles like legs, thighs, arms, calves, etc. Pregnant women have to be even more careful, as their ankles and the sides of their hips will naturally accumulate water during the course of the pregnancy. So if their body had excess water before they got pregnant, they will feel bloated and very uncomfortable during the pregnancy. Their breasts will swell up earlier than usual and more than normal, and so will their ankles and hips. So if you are planning a baby, you need to be even more vigilant, and make sure that your body does not have water retention. And if it does, it needs to be addressed before you get pregnant.

Another important reason for water retention is the intake of excess salt. Our bodies need only 2–3 grams of salt each day for normal functioning. But with our food habits, and the trend for quick ready-to-eat meals, we tend to cross that limit. Canned or tinned food, preserves, processed food, salad dressings, heavy mayonnaise and all readymade foods like packaged soups, curries, veggies, etc. have excess salt and should be avoided. In fact, you should try and replace normal salt with rock salt or sendha namak in your food whenever possible as it is low on the sodium content. These are simple solutions available around you, which you can

Tips for reducing salt intake

- Do not add extra salt in salads, fruits.
- Have saltless omelette, nimbu paani.
- Cabbage, spinach, and mushroom don't need salt; you can cook them with little or no salt.
- Chips, canned, tinned food, preserves, salad dressings, heavy mayonnaise; all readymade food have excess salt and should be avoided.
- Never have rice for dinner; it makes you feel heavy and turns into water during the night.
- Use more of rock salt or sendha namak which has less sodium than normal salt.

easily embrace. Also, avoid adding extra salt to your food, especially fruits and salads. You really don't need to. And eat things which have less or natural salt in them like cabbage, mushrooms, etc. Incorporate vegetables such as celery, onion, eggplant, asparagus, ginger, parsley, and watermelon, which are said to have a diuretic effect, into your diet. Excess salt is harmful even for people with high blood pressure, and needs to be controlled.

Effects of water retention

Our body reacts to excess water in several visible ways. These are telltale signs and a way for you to realize that you need to do something about it. The most common effects of water retention can be experienced in the weakening of the muscles and bones. Your muscles become sluggish and lose their natural strength. You might have often heard about some sportsmen being more prone to injuries than the rest. You can get muscle cramps easily with a higher risk of wear and tear in the body. If your bones get weakened, the first areas to get affected are your joints. In general, you will be more susceptible to sprains and aches in your body. You will feel tired soon, and if you press your muscles, you will feel a shooting pain. This will not be the case with a normal fit person.

In the long run, your internal organs also get affected, the result being that you are more prone to infections and other external attacks to your body. It can even lead to chronic problems like hypertension and high blood pressure. Your appetite flares up considerably, and there are more incidences of constipation. Both these factors make you pile on more kilos. So now you know, how drinking less water can make you put on weight.

For women, who experience bloating during their PMS, I have one simple advice: drink more water. One of the main causes of bloating before your periods is lack of sufficient water intake. I have a friend who used to have her periods like clockwork, bang on time. But recently, she started having irregular periods, and was really confused and worried. Guess what the cause was: drinking less water. So now you know how important water is for your body, especially if you want to lose weight. You just cannot ignore it!

Panipuri as a laxative

Did you know that your favourite panipuri works as an excellent laxative? Yes, it's true. Panipuri water contains mint, rock salt or kala namak, jeera, and coriander, which act as cooling agents for the stomach. They work like a natural laxative and help in your bowel movements, making your mornings happier. Panipuri cleans and clears the inner lining of the intestine, and is a natural remedy for constipation. Have two glasses of panipuri water if you have irregular bowels and experience the difference the next morning. People with stomach ulcers and urinary problems should, however, avoid this.

How to cure water retention?

It is as simple as it sounds: drink more water to cure water retention! You must drink at least 4–5 litres of water in a day. Try and store water in a copper vessel and drink it in silver glasses. It is an age-old remedy but still works wonders as it helps digestion, which in turn reduces water retention and weight gain. The first and foremost thing is to learn how to drink water. Just as you cannot have all your three meals together, you should not drink litres of water in one go, but drink it at regular intervals throughout the day. Here's a simple and practical routine that you can follow for drinking water:

My everyday water chart

- Have one bottle of regular water at room temperature when you wake up. People who are constipated can drink lukewarm water instead.
- 20 minutes after breakfast: 1 glass
- 1 glass before lunch
- After lunch: 1 glass
- 2 glasses of water 20 minutes before exercising
- During the workout sip water, do not gulp; water is used to lose weight; when the body gets too full; no cold water, only normal water
- 2–3 glasses after workout
- Carry a bottle of water (1 litre) in your bag; refill when done
- 1 glass before teatime
- 1 glass before dinner
- After dinner: 1 glass
- 1–2 glasses before sleeping

You can print this out and paste it on your fridge or near your workstation so that you can remember when and how to drink water. We are all slaves of habit. Just as we get into a habit of drinking less water, likewise we can make drinking the right amount of water a habit. This time is a good one to start!

Getting started

Rule one: Wear the right clothes and shoes

Before you start working out, be it any form of exercise, make sure that you are wearing the right kind of shoes and clothes. Take care to wear shoes that are well cushioned. Never run, jog, or exercise in your floaters, chappals, or even canvas shoes, as it can damage your joints. You should always run on a hard surface. In fact, a mud track is the best track to run on. You can even run on the beach, but on hard sand, not soft. Also, remember never to run or jog on concrete. As far as your clothing is concerned, it should be comfortable and stretchable, so avoid tight-fitting jeans or shirts.

Rule two: Don't exercise for more than 1½ hours at a time

You should ideally not exercise for more than 1½ hours at a stretch. I usually advise against it. You can exercise for more than 1½ hours in a day if you want to lose weight faster but only at intervals. Doing more is an overload on the body, and will only end up causing all kinds of sprains and aches. However, some workouts can be for a little less or more time than this, depending upon the kind of exercises. If you are doing it under the guidance of an expert then you don't need to worry about it. And as far as the frequency goes, you should exercise six days in a week. Take a break on the seventh day and just rest and relax. If you do not have time, vary your duration of exercise from 1 hour to 30 minutes. The days when you have to go out or are very busy due to any reason, you can exercise for only 30 minutes.

Rule three: Always stretch before and after exercising

Did you ever come back from a workout at a gym and could not move your arms or your legs? Most likely, this is the result of not stretching before or after your workout. When you are doing yoga, all your body parts open up and more blood flows into the muscles you are stretching. But when you are doing other forms of exercises, your body might end up getting stiff, if you do not stretch before and after your workout. Many gym goers, especially those who start working out after a gap, get muscle cramps and cannot move their arms, legs, shoulders, etc. Some of them don't stretch as they feel that the muscle that they were pumping and trying to bulk up would get back to its normal state. However, such people also need to stretch. What they can do is stretch the part, not the same day, but the next day—if they feel their muscles would get flaccid.

I have often seen how a lot of people underestimate the importance of stretching. But why is stretching so important? Stretching helps to relax and provide a shape to the body. What many people don't know is that it also plays an important role in losing weight. If you stretch regularly, you are less prone to injuries, aches, and pains. You feel more energetic and tend to recover faster than others. I can give you my own example here. The normal time for getting healed after a ligament tear is eight months but since I stretch regularly, I recovered in just one month. You must also remember not to bounce while stretching. Some common stretching exercises are; Sarpasana, for the stomach; Paschimottanasana, for the hamstrings on the back of the legs; Bhadrasana, for the hips, and Tadasana for the entire body.

These can be done by anybody for 30 seconds, in 3 sets.

1. Sarpasana: Lie down on the stomach with your forehead on the floor, hand by the side of the body, slowly bend both your elbows, bringing the palms close to the chest, with elbows facing upwards close to the body. Slowly inhale raising the head, shoulders, chest, and stomach till your navel region, with the help of the hands. In the final position, hold for 20 seconds with normal breathing and then slowly come down to the starting position. Repeat in 3 sets.

2. Paschimottanasana: Sit on the floor keeping your legs straight and palms on your thighs, keeping your heels on the floor. Inhale, taking your hands upwards with your palms facing each other. Now bend forward and try and get a hold of your foot with the help of your hands, without bending your knees, keep bending forward as much as you can while trying to touch your knees with your nose. Hold this position for 20 seconds breathing normally and then, slowly come back to the starting position. Repeat in 3 sets.

    Initially one may not be flexible enough to get into this posture, as the fats in the abdomen may act as a barrier. At the initial stage, bend as much as you can, but don't bend your knees. Don't do it too fast, as the important thing is to remain in the bending posture for a longer duration than to do it more and more randomly.

3.   Bhadrasana: Sit on the floor putting the soles of your feet together, hold your toes and slowly move your knees up and down a few times to loosen the inner thighs; then hold your feet with both hands and press your knees towards the floor and hold the position for 20 seconds while breathing normally, and then slowly come back to the normal position. Repeat in 3 sets.

4.   Tadasana: Stand straight with your feet shoulder width apart, with your hands to the side of your body. Inhale slowly raising your hands upwards with your palms facing each other and stretch your entire body while standing on your toes. Hold the final position for 20 seconds with normal breathing, and exhaling slowly come down to the starting position Repeat in 3 sets.

Rule four: Do not hold your breath while doing any exercise

I have noticed that many people do not breathe normally while exercising. It is very important to breathe normally and not hold your breath while exercising. You need to inhale and exhale regularly otherwise you will end up stressing all your internal organs. Whenever you get into any posture for an asana always make sure that you inhale while bending backward and exhale while bending forward. And when you get to your final posture breathe normally. When you disrupt your breathing, you apply extra pressure on your body, and can end up creating newer problems.

Don't work out with the air conditioner on!

A lot of people underestimate the importance of sweating while exercising, be it any form of exercise like yoga, aerobics, weight training, etc. This is because they want to lose weight and feel cool and comfortable at the same time. This is one thing that I feel very strongly about: you should never exercise with the air conditioner on. When you exercise with the airconditioner on, the body is still warm and supple while the outside environment is cool. There is a sharp difference in temperature, which leads to a very unhealthy clash preventing you from sweating. Also, your muscles respond better without an air conditioner, as they stretch better in normal room temperature. So if you workout without the air conditioner on, you can lose weight faster. On the other hand, if you keep your air conditioner on, your skin is still cool and you don't sweat enough. As a result, the excess salt remains trapped inside your body and cannot come out.

Also, people with asthma should especially make sure that they exercise in an open space or a non-air conditioner environment as this can aggravate their breathing problems. They keep on inhaling the stale air circulating in the room, which can further deteriorate their condition.

Rule five: Never workout during the first three days of your periods

Listen up all women! This is a rule especially for you. You should never exercise during the first three days of your periods. I genuinely feel that you should give your body rest during this time, at least for three days. This is a time for your body to be pampered, and by exercising during this time, you will only harm your body.

Let's begin

One of the things that I love about my job is that I get to meet
different kinds of people—housewives, working professionals,
wannabe stars, socialites, and celebrities. And they do leave
me amused at times. Radha Sen was eighty-eight kilos at 5 feet
8 inches, single, and a vegetarian. She had just crossed thirty-
five years and already had various kinds of medical problems
like asthma, PCOD, and joint pain. Radha was obese, being
around twenty-two kilos overweight, and she wanted to lose
all of that weight in a month! Believe me, this is true. And
there are many more Radhas around. In fact, this is one of the
most common requests that I get all the time. Can I get slim
in a month? What do I need to do to get to my normal weight
in a month? Most of these women are really impatient and
want to lose weight because they are getting married, have to
attend some wedding or family function, want to fit into the
black dress for the Christmas or for the New Year bash, etc.
My reply to them is simple: if you put on all this weight in a
month you surely will lose it in the same time. We all need to
understand that fitness is not a one month punishment but a
lifelong gift. It is like a habit that you need to cultivate.

Women after they cross thirty tend to put on weight around
their stomach, thighs, hips, etc., and they really need to be
conscious of this fact. Also, the most common time during the
year to put on weight is Diwali, the summer holidays between
May to June, and finally around Christmas and New Year's
Eve. These are what I call the 'red months', when you need to
be extra careful and exert more self-control than usual. Even
if you eat sweets, cakes, and other delicacies, never forget to
workout, and in greater frequency, to maintain your body.

Being in the fitness industry for so many years, I can now almost guess how many kilos overweight a person is just by looking at them. But that, I believe, comes only with experience. And by now even you would know how many kilos overweight you are and how many kilos you need to shed. I have always felt that it is easier to work with a goal in mind. Once you know the number of kilos you need to shed to look slim and sexy, it will give you the necessary drive to work hard. We have also talked at length about how to exercise, and what all to keep in mind to get the best results.

Before I prescribe any workout, we need to keep in mind the person's age, gender, BMI, medical history, injuries, lifestyle, how they put on weight, if they have ever worked out in their lives or not, are they vegetarian or non vegetarian, etc. I then look at their face, arms, upper body, lower body, body type—whether they are stiff or flabby—and so on to assess the person's body. I then make them do some basic exercises to test their flexibility, strength, endurance, etc. Based on all this I develop a specific exercise regime that will work best for them.

I am now going to share with you the exercise routines I have learnt over time and with experience. The yoga workouts that you will come across in this book are all different combinations of kriyas, asanas, Pranayam, and cardio-vascular exercises. Let me introduce you to them briefly so that you understand what you are doing, better.

Kriyas

These are basically cleansing techniques for the body that help to throw toxins and impurities out of the body, thereby keeping you rejuvenated. Kriyas relax the muscles, reduce fatigue, and help control the mucus from the internal organs. In the long run, they help find a balance between the mental and the emotional sides of our personality, which is crucial in today's times. Kriyas also clear acne, relieve migraines and, if done regularly, bring about a glow on the skin. The kriyas that I find most useful and often use in my regimes are:

- Jalneti kriya—clears the nasal passage
- Vaman kriya—removes excess mucus and indigested particles from the stomach
- Shankhaprakshalana kriya (under supervision only)— cleans the intestines
- Kapalbhati kriya—tones the internal organs such as the liver, stomach, spleen, kidney, colon, etc.

Asanas

Asanas are yoga postures that work on the organ or organs that they are designed for. They first affect the internal organs of the body, and the results consequently show on the external parts in the form of enhanced flexibility, toned muscles and a disease free body. Asanas help in the secretion of juices in the glands, aid better functioning of the excretory, hormonal, digestive, nervous, and other systems. The circulation of blood to all the parts of the body improves with asanas, which in turn brings about a radiant glow to the face. If you hold the asanas for a minute or more, then over time, it helps in the development of cells, increases concentration, self-confidence, self-restraint, etc. The asanas also relieve fatigue in the body and keep it active. There are many asanas that I have used in the book for different purposes. What matters is how you do them and the combination in which you use them.

Pranayam

Pranayam is a controlled breathing technique, which brings about calmness and stability as it works as a bridge between the mind and the body. It reduces the wear and tear of the body, lowers blood pressure, and relaxes the body against tension, which in turn results in calmer nerves. When the breathing is slow and deep, it covers all the parts of the body, which again distributes an equal amount of energy, through the blood circulation, to all the areas. This is something that does not happen with regular breathing! I have commonly used Pranayams such as Bhastrika, Anulom Vilom, and Bhramari in my workouts.

In this chapter, I have taken up four specific case studies for four specific weight issues that I come across most commonly—three for losing weight and one for putting on weight—and suggested workout regimes for them. If you fall in any of these categories, you too can follow the suggested regime, to address your weight issues. Unless you have a specific problem, these regimes should work for you too. I have illustrated most of these asanas with the help of photographs at the end of the chapter. Try and match your posture as close as possible to the pictures when you perform these asanas as it does make a difference.

For best results undertake the following basic precautions:
1. Never workout on a heavy stomach.
2. Exercise preferably 2 hours after your breakfast and 4 hours after your lunch.

3. When you start following the workouts, there is a possibility that you may, initially, feel a certain amount of dizziness. This is very common among people who do not exercise regularly. This happens due to the toxins that are eliminated from the body in the form of sweat. However, your body should ideally get accustomed to the asanas by two weeks from the time you start exercising.

4. Soreness in the body is also something that you might experience, in the beginning of your workouts, as you might not have stretched your body in a long time. Here again, you do not need to worry as your body should adapt to the workout in two weeks.

5. All the asanas in this book have to be performed in the given sequence, for them to have the desired effect on your body.

6. It is very important to know how to breathe while doing the asanas. You need to inhale while getting into a posture in which you have to bend backwards, exhale when you are bending forward, and then breathe normally while holding a posture.

7. Focus on the muscle or area that is getting affected while doing a particular posture.

8. There should be a break of at least 10 seconds between each asana.

9. Stretch before and after the exercises, even if it is for a few minutes.

10. Never overstretch the body while doing any asana and do it with absolute ease, focusing on your breathing.

11. After any workout, maintain a gap of 45 minutes before having any food.
12. For best results, eat a balanced diet at regular intervals to avoid constipation and indigestion.
13. Drink at least four to five litres of water in a day.

Case study 1: When you are five to ten kilos overweight

Radhika Singhania, a 31-year-old woman, delivered a baby girl four months ago, through a normal delivery. She is a socialite and it was important for her to lose weight as her appearance means a lot to her. An attractive woman at 5 feet 5 inches, Radhika has a medium frame. She goes out for lunches and dinners frequently, and even likes to party, so she wanted to get back into shape as soon as possible.

Radhika came to me for help to lose her excess pregnancy weight, which she was finding very difficult to shed. At the time she walked into my studio, she weighed seventy-six kilos. When we got talking, she told me that during her pregnancy, she had put on twenty-five kilos, of which she had managed to lose fifteen but was just not able to shed the last eight to ten kilos. She was feeding her baby and losing a bit of weight due to that, but not as much as, and as quickly as, she wanted. Keeping in mind her body frame and lifestyle, I planned an easy to do and practical regime for Radhika. Her goal was to lose at least eight kilos, and we aimed to lose it in four months. Due to Radhika's dedication, she managed to lose eight kilos in three months and a total of eleven kilos in four months. If you too are five to ten kilos overweight or have had a baby recently, you can follow the same regime. Women with normal delivery can follow this routine after three months of delivery, but women who have undergone a C-section should start only after four months.

Radhika's regime

Where: Choose a place which has fresh air circulation, preferably a garden, a terrace, or a workout place in your house. In Radhika's case, she came to my studio for her workouts.

What you need for the asanas: A yoga mat, a bottle of water, and a hand or face towel. You can also play some nice slow music in the background if you like.

Warming up before the asanas: Spread the mat on the floor and sit in a comfortable position. Take five to ten long breaths to relax yourself, then lie down on your back and stretch yourself by raising your hands up and toes downward about five times.

1st week

Walk for 20 minutes, normally and leisurely, three days a week. Radhika walked on the treadmill at my studio at 4 km/hr.

2nd week

Walk for 20 minutes, normally and leisurely, six days a week. Radhika used to walk on the beach.

3rd week

Walk for 30 minutes normally, three days a week. Walk for 45 minutes, alternating between 5 minutes fast, then 10 minutes normally, three days a week. In Radhika's case, she walked on the treadmill at 5.5 km/hr (fast) and 4.5 km/hr (slow).

4th week

For the fourth week, the total walking time per day should be 45 minutes. Walk fast for 5 minutes, then normally for 10 minutes, six days a week. Here, Radhika would alternate between the beach and the treadmill. The days she could not make it to my studio due to any reason, she would simply take a walk on the beach. By the end of four weeks Radhika had lost two kilos. She was feeling energetic and fresh. In the first two weeks, she found even walking difficult but at the end of four weeks, as her body started feeling lighter, she felt ready to get into a slightly tougher routine.

5th week

In the 5th week, I introduced simple yoga exercises for her. These set of exercises needed to be done three times a week. We started with some basic stretching and slow body movements.

Warm up for 5–6 minutes: stretch every body part starting from the neck; neck rotations, shoulder rotations, sideway movements for back, arms, and stomach; hip rotations, lunging downwards for the lower body with one leg forward and one leg back. I then made her do some standing asanas to check her fitness level.

Hold each standing asana for 15 seconds; one set each:
- Trikonasana
- Tadasana
- Side bending Chakrasana

Then we did some sitting asanas. I made her hold each sitting asana for 15 seconds; one set each:

- Vakrasana
- Ustrasana
- Supta Vajrasana
- Paschimottanasana

The sitting asanas made Radhika feel good and energetic. These were followed by some asanas in the supine position. Lie down on your back and hold each of these asanas for 15 seconds; one set each

- Pavanmuktasana
- Ek Pada Ardha Halasana (coordination)
- Naukasana

Then we did some postures lying on the stomach. Hold each of these asanas in prone position for 15 seconds; one set each:

- Bhujangasana
- Sarpasana
- Ardha Shalabhasana
- Dhanurasana

After these asanas, I made Radhika relax in Shavasana for 10 minutes to relax her entire body. Then I made her sit in Sukhasana, a comfortable position, where you keep your back straight and relax your facial muscles. It was her first week of yoga exercises, so I decided to make her do some easy breathing exercises like:

- Sahaja Pranayam: 3 rounds
- Kapalbhati kriya: 50 strokes, 1 round
- Brahma Mudra: 3 rounds
- Om chanting or any auspicious chant—3 times

On the other three days during the 5th week, you can walk for a total of 45 minutes, alternating between 5 minutes normal and 5 minutes fast. Radhika walked on the treadmill at 5.5 km/hr (fast) and 4.5 km/hr (slow).

6th week

For the 6th week, Radhika repeated the asanas she did in the 5th week. However, instead of 1 set, I increased it to 2 sets each, four days a week. On the rest of the two days, she walked on the treadmill at 5.5 km/hr (fast) and 4.5 km/hr (slow) just as she did during the 5th week.

7th and 8th week

In the 7th week I made Radhika do the same asanas as in the 6th week, but increased the time duration from 15 to 25 seconds, 2 sets each.

Increased the walking time to 1 hour, two days a week, alternating between 5 minutes slow and 5 minutes fast. Radhika walked on the treadmill at 6 km/hr (fast) and 5 km/ hr (slow) for the same time duration.

At the end of the 8th week, Radhika had lost another three kilos. So, all together, she lost five kilos in two months alongwith many inches. **I have often noticed that the last three to five kilos are the most difficult to shed as people usually tend to get complacent.** They start fitting into their old clothes and feel really happy about it. But it is really important to keep yourself motivated by concentrating on your actual goal, and keep on working hard irrespective of small successes. So in this case since Radhika wanted to get down to sixty-three kilos, I kept on reminding her that this is only half of what she wanted and that she was yet to reach the finishing line!

9th and 10th week

For the 9th week, we concentrated on brisk movements. Radhika would first warm up for 5 to 8 minutes every time before starting a session. I then made her do 10 rounds of slow Suryanamaskars. This was followed by the asanas listed below for 25 seconds, one set each:

Standing positions:

- Trikonasana + 1 round of Suryanamaskar
- Tadasana + 1 round of Suryanamaskar
- Ardha Chandrasana + 1 round of Suryanamaskar
- Side bending Chakrasana + 1 round of Suryanamaskar

That was the week in which I introduced a few new sitting positions:

- Vakrasana
- Akarna Dhanurasana
- Paschimottanasana
- Ugrasana
- Ustrasana

Supine positions:

- Pavanmuktasana

- Naukasana variations
- Setubandhasana

Prone positions:
- Triyak Bhujangasana
- Naukasana
- Dhanurasana
- Makarasana for relaxation
- Sharnagat Mudra in sitting position or Vajrasana
- Brahma Mudra: 2 rounds
- Chandrabedhan: 10 rounds
- Kapalbhati: 50 strokes, 3 rounds each
- Om chanting or any auspicious chant: 5 rounds

At the end, Radhika sat for 2 minutes in meditation focusing on her normal breathing pattern.

On the other two days, Radhika walked briskly for an hour on the beach as she enjoys fresh air.

11th and 12th week

Repeat all the asanas done in the 9th and 10th week but increase it to 2 sets each. Also, walk briskly for 1 hour two days a week.

By now, Radhika had lost another three kilos and some more inches. She was taking a balanced diet and exercising regularly without missing out a single day, except the three days she had her periods. At the end of three months, Radhika had lost eight kilos in all.

Zoa's exercise routine

Age: 22   Weight: 46 kilos   Sessions: 1 hour, six days a week
Target: Zoa Morani is now slim and energetic. She started with losing weight but now her goal is to maintain her weight and stay fit.

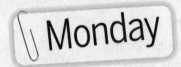

Monday

Monday is the beginning of the week and on this day we focus on the upper body— so most of the exercises below work on areas such as arms, stomach, and back.

1 Warm up with some body stretching
2 Suryanamaskar: 25 rounds
    Relax for 2 minutes

Prone positions:

3 Santolanasana: facing the ground with elbows bent hold for 20 seconds, then 25 push-ups
4 Bhujangasana and Konasana (position number 7 to 8 of Suryanamaskar): 20 times

Supine positions:

5 Ardha Naukasana (lift your upper body supporting your neck with your hands): 20 seconds

6 Ardha Halasana (lifting both legs 45 to 90 degrees to the floor): 20 seconds
7 Naukasana (lifting upper and lower body together): 20 seconds

Repeat these sets of exercises four times. The following asanas are for the arms and the stomach:

8 Kati Chakrasana or the crocodile pose: 4 times

Sitting position

9 Gomukhasana (cow pose): 2 times

The following exercises help her to relax:

10 Shavasana: 5 minutes
11 Kapalbhati kriya: 200 strokes
12 Anulom Vilom Pranayam: 4 rounds
13 Bhastrika Pranayam: 5 rounds

{ Yoga has been my greatest discovery till date. The energy and strength it has given me mentally and physically has been phenomenal. Always include a fitness regime into your lifestyle that you love and enjoy doing. }

Tuesday

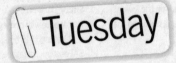

On Tuesday we concentrate on postures and do a few of cardiovascular exercises.

1 Warm up with stretches
2 Suryanamaskar: 25 rounds
3 10 Suryanamaskars while repeating position numbers 5, 6, 7, three times in 1 round of Suryanamaskar to stretch the arms and abdominal muscles

Standing positions:

4 Side bending Chakrasana: hold for 15 seconds, 3 sets
5 Natarajasana: hold for 20 second, 3 sets
6 Trikonasana: hold for 20 second, 3 sets

Supine positions:

7 Sarvanganasana: hold for 20 seconds, 3 sets

8 Chakrasana: hold for 15 seconds, 3 sets
9 Pavanmuktasana: hold for 20 seconds, 2 sets

Prone positions:

10 Bhujangasana: hold for 20 seconds, 2 sets
11 Makarasana: hold for 30 seconds, 1 set

Sitting positions:

12 Paschimottanasana: hold for 20 seconds, 2 sets
13 Vakrasana: hold for 20 seconds, 2 sets

Pranayam

14 Anulom Vilom: 5 rounds
15 Sheetali Pranayam: 10 rounds
16 Shavasana: 5 minutes

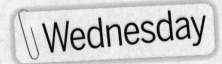

Wednesday

On Wednesday, we work on the lower body and target the legs, butt, and the sides.

1 Warm up with stretches
2 Suryanamaskar: 25 rounds
   Take a break and relax for 5 minutes.

Standing positions:
3 Chair pose: hold for 20 seconds, then 25 times sit-ups
4 Raise on toes: hold for 20 seconds, then heels up and down 25 times
5 Tadasana: hold for 20 seconds, 10 times
6 Side bending Chakrasana: hold for 20 seconds, 15 times on both the sides

Sitting positions:
7 Cat pose with one leg raised up: hold for 20 seconds, 15 times, both legs
8 Paschimottanasana: hold for 10 seconds, 2 times

Supine position:
9 Poorna Halasana: hold for 10 seconds

Prone position:
10 Dhanurasana: hold for 10 seconds

The following exercises help her to relax:
11 Makarasana: hold for 1 minute
12 Ujjayi Pranayam: 5 rounds
13 Om chanting: 3 times

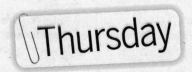

Thursday

Thursday is the day for kriyas, as by now we have covered almost all body parts.

1 Start with normal warm up and stretches
2 Kapalbhati: 200 strokes
3 Jalneti: 2 rounds with each nostril
4 Kapalbhati: 200 strokes
5 Vaman kriya: 1 round
6 Kapalbhati: 100 strokes
7 Pada Hastasana to reduce the water in the nostrils for 20 seconds 3 rounds
8 Brahma Mudra: 10 seconds on each side, 2 sets
9 Bhramari Pranayam: 10 rounds
10 Shavasana: 10 minutes

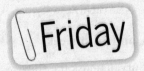

Friday

On the last working day of the week, we do cardio vascular exercises and target the entire body.

1 Warm up with full body stretches
2 Suryanamaskar: 25 rounds
   Take a break of 2 minutes after this
3 Spot jogging 15 second + 10 sit ups, Suryanamaskar, 10 times
   Take a break for 2 minutes
4 Suryanamaskar with 5 push ups, 10 times
   Take a break for 2 minutes

Standing positions:
5 Ardha Halasana: hold for 10 seconds, 2 times
6 Natarajasana: hold for 10 seconds, 2 times
7 Hanuman asana: hold for 10 seconds, 2 times
8 Parvatasana: hold for 10 seconds, 2 times

Sitting positions:
9 Ustrasana: hold for 10 seconds, 2 times
10 Matsyendrasana: hold for 10 seconds, 2 times

Supine positions:
11 Naukasana: hold for 10 seconds, 2 times
12 Chakrasana: hold for 10 seconds, 2 times

Prone positions:
13 Sarpasana: hold for 10 seconds, 2 times
14 Poorna Shalabhasana: hold for 10 seconds, 2 times

The following exercises help her to relax:
15 Makarasana: hold for 1 minute
16 Chandra Bhedan Pranayam: 5 times
18 Sheetali Pranayam: 5 times

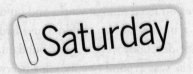

Saturday

Stretching
On Saturdays we do only stretches and no Suryanamaskars due to the hectic workout of the previous day.

13th, 14th, 15th, and 16th week

Do 20 rounds of Suryanamaskars, slowly.

Repeat the asanas of the 11th and 12th week but increase it to 3 sets each.

Walk briskly for 1 hour; 2 times a week. Here again, Radhika chose to walk on the beach.

By the end of this routine, Radhika had lost about eleven kilos in total and achieved what she had set out to do. She was down to fifty-seven kilos and still losing weight. It's been four months now since we started working and Radhika feels very energetic and fresh, and is a very confident mother of a year-old-baby. Interestingly, she looks even better than before. Her body has undergone a structural change. In fact, she feels so nice that she is ready to try for another baby as she feels that it is easy getting back into shape.

Case study 2: When you are ten to twenty kilos overweight

I still remember Sheetal Oberoi who came to me very depressed, not knowing what to do. At 5 feet 3 inches, she weighed seventy-six kilos. And although she was medically fit at forty years, she did not stick to a disciplined or routine lifestyle. There was no fixed time of work, and no time to eat or sleep. She was a mother of two children and had to travel a lot for work. Her ideal body weight was around fifty-four to fifty-eight kilos so she was around twenty kilos overweight. Sheetal was not overweight but obese. Due to her weight, she was really stressed out and had regular complaints of constipation.

Sheetal had not done rigorous exercise or played any sport. However, she did like to walk. So I didn't want to give her anything drastic, especially since she had crossed 40 and was not as young and flexible as before. In fact, for anybody over forty, it is not advisable to start exercising strenuously, or play any new and exhausting sport, as it may do more harm than good. You might end up injuring your knees and other joints as a result. For such people, it is always better to start with something that the body is accustomed to. So I asked Sheetal to start working out slowly and gradually keeping in mind her age and fitness level. We started out with walking, followed by Suryanamaskars, as she had done these before and was comfortable with these. I followed this with other basic exercises and devised a daily exercise routine for her.

Sheetal's routine

Where: Choose a place which has fresh air circulation preferably a garden, a terrace, or a workout place in your house.

What you need for the asanas: A yoga mat, a bottle of water, and a hand or face towel. You can also play some nice slow music in the background if you like.

Warming up: Spread the mat on the floor and sit in a comfortable position. Take five to ten long breaths to relax yourself, then lie on your back and stretch yourself by raising your hands up and toes downward about five times.

1st week

- 20 minutes of brisk walking as she was used to it already
- Kapalbhati: 50 strokes, 3 rounds
- Ardha Halasana: hold at 90 degrees, 5 seconds on

each side, 20 sets

- Ardha Naukasana: for the upper body, hold for 20 seconds, 3 sets

2nd week

For the 2nd week, repeat the exercises as in the 1st week. Also, include Suryanamaskars, 15 rounds.

3rd week

For the 3rd week, Sheetal did 20 minutes of walking on the treadmill, alternating between 5 minutes slow, at 4.5 km/hr, then 2 minutes running at 6 km/hr, in 3 sets.

- Kapalbhati: 50 strokes, 10 sets
- Naukasana: 20 times
- Suryanamaskar: 30 rounds
- Bhujangasana: hold for 10 seconds, 3 sets
- Dhanurasana: hold for 10 seconds, 3 sets
- Sarpasana: hold for 10 seconds, 3 sets

4th week

- Spot jogging: 2 minutes
- Kapalbhati: 100 strokes while standing, 3 sets
- 20 Suryanamaskars: 2 rounds, slowly
- Naukasana: hold for 15 seconds, 10 sets
- Side bending Chakrasana: hold for 10 seconds, 5 sets
- Dhanurasana: hold for 10 seconds, 5 sets
- Bhujangasana: hold for 10 seconds, 5 sets
- Bhastrika Pranayam: 5 rounds, 20 strokes Kapalbhati + 1 round Anulom Vilom = 1 round Bhastrika

- Bhramari Pranayam: 10 rounds
- Shavasana: 5 minutes

At the end of one month Sheetal had lost five kilos. She continued this routine for four months and by the end of it she had lost 25 inches and fifteen kilos. Today she loves herself and has realized how important it is to look after your body. She continues to workout and has started enjoying her job better than before. Her stress levels are under check, and the recurring constipation too has long since bid adieu. Sheetal Oberoi is happy today after achieving what she had set out to do.

Case study 3: When you are twenty to forty kilos overweight or overly obese

Ruby Shroff is 25 years old, 5 feet 2 inches in height, and weighed ninty-nine kilos. She works for an MNC and is not married. Due to her excessive obesity, she had developed other health problems like indigestion, and lower-back ache. Ruby had tried very hard to lose weight, but nothing seemed to be working for her. When she finally came to me, she had done all kinds of things from going to the gym, doing aerobics and following anorexic diets. Initially, she did lose a little weight but then gained back many more kilos. Ruby had also been experiencing excessive hair loss, and she used to be constantly irritated about everything.

Finally she got my number from a friend and called me. She sounded desperate and said that I was her last hope. I told her that it was possible for her to lose weight but she did not seem to believe me. When I met Ruby, I felt she was pretty but had given up on herself. She looked dejected and stressed out.

I want to tell all the Rubys of the world that it is indeed possible to lose weight, and that you should never give up hope. My challenge was to make her lose weight and make her look the way she had long dreamed of. I really wanted her to succeed. In such cases, we have to focus on all aspects of the body. I like to start with finding out the root cause of the problem, so I decided to first put her on a cleansing programme instead of an exercise routine. Cleansing in yoga refers to clearing up the blockages in the body.

1. I made her do Jalneti and Sutraneti to clear the nasal passage. This also improves the blood circulation and opens up all the blockages mental and physical.
2. She then cleaned her stomach through Vaman kriya.
3. Her intestine was cleared through Shankprakshalan.

We started with Jalneti and Vaman daily and Shankprak-shalan once a week. I told her not to eat any junk food, but only regular healthy home-cooked food. After two weeks of doing these cleansing kriyas, Ruby started sharing her problems with me. She told me that she had PCOD (polycystic ovarian disease), which believe it or not is one of the most common causes of infertility in women nowadays. Now my aim to give her a healthy and slim body came up against another challenge, as it is very difficult for women with PCOD to lose weight.

Ruby's routine

I started doing yoga with Ruby in the 4th week after her body had been cleansed with the help of the kriyas. I did not want her to venture straight into strenuous workouts as she had never worked out regularly before and this could damage her body, causing injuries. The cleansing process was also important as by now she was mentally prepared for the workout and the asanas, would have the best results on her body.

Where: Choose a place which has fresh air circulation, preferably a garden, a terrace, or a workout place in your house.

What you need for the asanas: A yoga mat, a bottle of water, and a hand or face towel. You can also play some nice slow music in the background if you like.

Warming up: Spread the mat on the floor and sit in a comfortable position. Take five to ten long breaths to relax yourself, then lie down on your back and stretch yourself by raising your hands up and toes downward about five times.

4th week

- Jalneti kriya
- Vaman kriya
- Kapalbhati: 500 strokes
- Warm up: start exercising for 5–6 minutes; stretch every body part starting from the neck. Neck rotations, shoulder rotations, sideways movements for back, arms, and stomach, lunging downwards for the lower body with one leg forward one leg back.
- Spot walking for 2 minutes
- Normal stretches for the arms, legs, chest, and back.

- Postures like Ardha Halasana, Bhujangasana, Poorna Shalabhasana, and Vakrasana, all for 10 seconds each
- Chandrabhedan Pranayam: 10 rounds

Ruby lost four kilos in four weeks but I felt she should have lost six kilos. I was feeling a little disappointed and it made me think that there was something else stopping her from losing weight. So I asked her to get a thyroid test done. As I had guessed, she tested positive for thyroid. This was an added challenge for me, as it is again very difficult for people with thyroid to lose weight. But we kept our fingers crossed and continued working together.

5th week

- 20 minutes slow walking on the treadmill at 4.5 km/hr
- Warm up exercises
- 10 Suryanamaskars
- 1 Suryanamaskar with 50 strokes of Kapalbhatis, 10 rounds
- 1 Suryanamaskar with 10 sit-ups, 10 rounds
- Naukasana on your back: hold for 5 seconds, 10 sets
- Naukasana on your stomach: hold for 10 seconds, 5 sets
- Ujjayi Pranayam in which you only exhale: 6 rounds

6th week

- 20 minutes of walking on the treadmill at 5km/hr
- Warm up exercises
- 10 Suryanamaskars
- 1 Suryanamaskar with 50 strokes of Kapalbhatis, 10 rounds

- 1 Suryanamaskar with 10 sit-ups, 10 rounds
- Naukasana on your back: hold for 10 seconds, 5 sets
- Naukasana on your stomach: hold for 15 seconds, 5 sets
- Ujjayi Pranayam in which you only exhale, 10 rounds
- Poorna Halasana with both legs: hold for 20 to 25 seconds, 4 sets
- Anulom Vilom Pranayam: 10 rounds

7th week

- 20 minutes slow walking on the treadmill at 5.05 km/hr
- Warm up exercises
- Suryanamaskars: 10 rounds
- 1 Suryanamaskar with 50 strokes Kapalbhatis, 10 rounds
- 1 Suryanamaskar with 10 sit-ups, 10 rounds
- Naukasana on your back: hold for 15 seconds, 5 sets
- Naukasana on your stomach: hold for 20 seconds, 5 sets
- Ujjayi Pranayam in which you only exhale: 10 rounds
- Poorna Halasana with both the legs: hold for 25 seconds, 5 sets
- Anulom Vilom Pranayam: 10 rounds
- Chair pose: hold for 5 seconds, 20 sets
- Ardha Chandrasana: hold for 15 seconds, 5 sets
- Standing sideways Chakrasana: hold for 15 seconds, 5 sets
- Dhanurasana on the stomach: hold for 10 seconds, 3 sets

8th week

As we had already done different kinds of exercises in the 7th week, I decided it was now time to check Ruby's strength, stamina and flexibility. I was interested in seeing whether Ruby was only losing weight or if she was improving on other aspects of fitness as well. For me overall fitness is very important, as with fitness weight loss is long lasting and does not make you feel weak or tired.

- Start with spot jogging for 10 minutes
- 50 Suryanamaskars in 2 sets
- Hold all postures for at least 30 seconds, 1 set each
- 1000 strokes of Kapalbhati in 2 rounds
- Chandrabhedan Pranayam: 10 rounds
- Ujjayi Pranayam: 10 rounds
- Om chanting or any auspicious chant: 5 rounds
- Shavasana: 5 minutes

Ruby lost ten kilos in eight weeks. Not only that, her PCOD came down by 40 per cent, thyroid by 60 per cent, and she no longer had any complaint of constipation. She was eating home-cooked meals at regular intervals and drinking four litres of water every day. Ruby had also started enjoying a regular good night's sleep. After six months of working out with me, she had lost twenty-six kilos and 40 inches all over the body. Ruby continues to work out and now has a healthy body and a stronger control over her mind. Although she is seventy-three kilos now, she is still working out to reach her ideal body weight, which is around fifty three to fifty-six kilos.

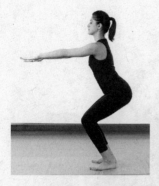

Utkatasana level 1
(chair pose)

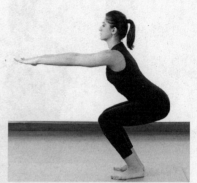

Utkatasana level 2
(chair pose)

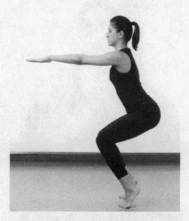

Utkatasana level 3
(chair pose)

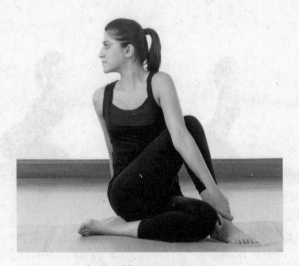

Ardha Matsyendrasana

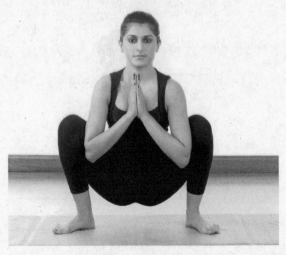

Naman Uttanasana

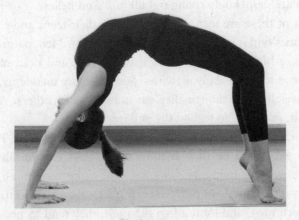

Chakrasana

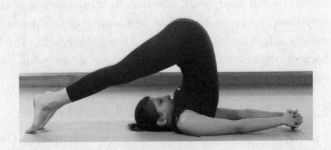

Poorna Halasana

Are you underweight?

While most of us are busy losing weight, there are some others who are desperately trying to bulk up. And believe it or not, most of these are men. A lot of men in their teens and early twenties find it very difficult to put on weight. Men, naturally have, a higher metabolic rate than women, and need more calories for their daily activities. Such men are unable to put on weight even though they eat normally like others. As a result, they end up feeling shy and frustrated.

Being skinny has a significant social impact as well. Thin men get teased by their friends, family, and are considered to be weak or unmanly. Girls, too, don't like very thin men, and prefer athletic or beefy ones. It affects the social relations of such men, and more often than not, they tend to become shy, diffident, and introverted. They hate to go out and meet people, always very conscious of the way they look or what others might think of them. So you know, there are all kinds of people. Some want to lose weight while there are others who are desperately trying to gain weight. You can be underweight due to many reasons such as high-metabolic rate, quantity and quality of food, work schedule. In many cases, it is also hereditary. I have noticed that men start putting on weight more easily, after they cross the 25-year threshold. This is because the metabolic rate keeps going down with each passing year.

Case study 4: When you are underweight

I get a lot of queries from men who are underweight. Only recently, my client Prithvi Bansal, who is a 20-year-old student called me to help him put on weight. Although he is 5 feet

11 inches in height, he weighs just fifty-three kilos. Prithvi used to be teased in college by his friends, as he was a really thin boy. I advised him to start exercising, but stop doing any cardio vascular exercises such as running or weight training. Prithvi wanted to put on ten to fifteen kilos, and I designed a basic workout routine for him accordingly. Alongside, I also asked him to start having more of foods which have proteins like eggs, meat, fish, and extra fruits like two to four bananas, chiku, apple, milk and milk products like paneer, cheese, cream, lassi, and butter. It is also advisable to drink water 30 minutes after having your food. It's been three months, and he has already put on four kilos, and waiting to pile on more!

A basic workout for putting on weight

Where: Choose a place which has fresh air circulation preferably a garden, a terrace, or a workout place in your house.

What you need for the asanas: A yoga mat, a bottle of water, and a hand or face towel. You can also play some nice slow music in the background if you like.

Warming up: Spread the mat on the floor and sit in a comfortable position. Take five to ten long breaths to relax yourself, then lie down on your back and stretch yourself by raising your hands upwards and toes downward about five times.

Do some light and easy postures three days a week:

- Ek Pada Halasana: hold for 20 seconds, 1 set
- Ardha Naukasana: hold 15 seconds
- Ardha Pavanmuktasana: hold 20 seconds, 1 set
- Kati Chakrasana: hold for 15 seconds, 1 set on each side
- Ardha Shalabhasana: hold for 15 seconds, 1 set with

each leg
- Bhujangasana: hold for 15 seconds, 1 set
- Paschimottanasana: hold for 15 seconds, 1 set
- Vakrasana: hold for 15 seconds, 1 set
- Parvatasana in Padmasana: hold for 15 seconds, 1 set
- Tadasana: hold 15 seconds, 10 times

Pranayam

- Anulom Vilom: 5 rounds
- Bhramari: 5 rounds

For relaxing at the end of the session:
- Shavasana: 15 minutes

Cheat tips for overweight women

- Wear corset bras if you want to make your chest and belly look thin.
- Wear high heels; it actually adds length and makes you look thinner.
- Wear loose clothes that hide the bulges and give you a uniform look.

Cheat tips for underweight men

- Wear loose clothes; never opt for body hugging clothes.
- Don't wear half sleeves.
- If you have really spindly legs, wear 2–3 tights below your trousers.

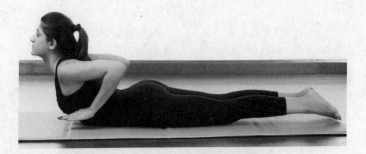

Bhujangasana

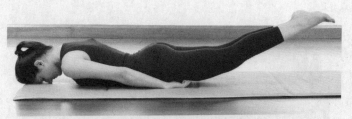

Poorna Shalabhasana

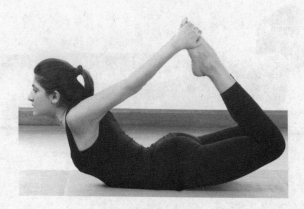

Dhanurasana

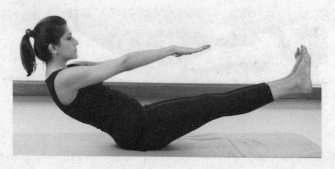

Naukasana (on the back)

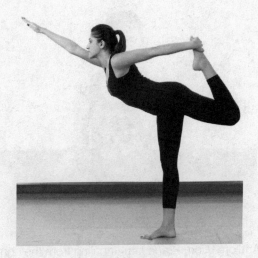

Natrajasana

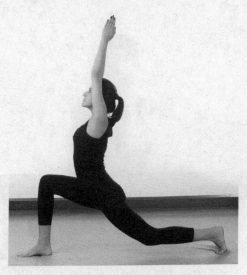

Ardha Chandrasana

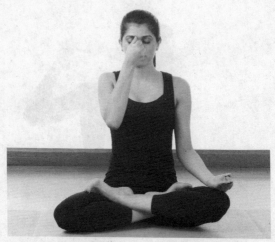

Anulom Vilom Pranayam (inhaling from the right)

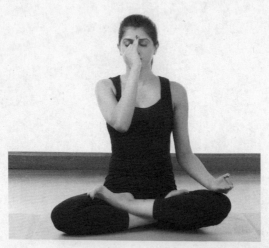

Anulom Vilom Pranayam (inhaling from the left)

2

How to become a perfect ten

When I met Payal almost five years ago, I was sixty-one kilos, and really frustrated. I have a naturally broad frame, and have always had to watch my weight. I had tried many things to lose weight like dieting, gyming, etc., but nothing seemed to be working. I love to eat, and depriving my body of food really made me feel even more depressed. I am a proper Punjabi girl who likes her paranthas, dals, etc., so I could not starve myself to lose weight.

Then I met Payal. I have been doing yoga with her for almost five years now, and the results are for everyone to see. Payal has not only helped me lose weight but has also changed the shape of my body. I have a slim and toned physique now. She also taught me how to work on my weak areas like my arms and my calves, where I was prone to put on weight. I lost many kilos with Payal's help in a year and then during *Tashan*, I lost a few more kilos to look sizzling for the role. Not only that, I now have a perfect ten body. So I am no longer the broad-shaped Punjabi girl that I was, and I can wear anything without thinking twice, be it Indian, western, fusion, or even a bikini.

I am always bikini ready and so can you be!

Kareena Kapoor

Almost five years ago, just after *Don* was released, I got a call from Kareena Kapoor. I felt nervous as well as excited when she said that she wanted to meet me.

When I reached her flat the next day, I was wondering what exactly she wanted from me. How would she behave? What would she think of me? What would she be wearing? Would she be rude or polite? Brushing these thoughts aside, when I finally rang the bell, the very gorgeous Kareena Kapoor herself opened the door.

'Hi Payal, how are you?' she said casually and politely. 'Come on in.'

As we got chatting, Kareena told me plainly. 'I don't like to do yoga but I have been told it really works.'

'Yes, it does. But what exactly are you looking for?' I asked a little surprised, not expecting her to be so frank in the first meeting.

'I want to lose weight, but my problem is that I love to eat. I'm a typical Punjabi kudi with a broad structure and even though I exercise almost every day, I don't seem to be getting the kind of results I want. And like everybody else, I too have my weak spots, where I tend to put on weight in a jiffy. So now I want to try something different.'

'Let's start and see how it goes,' I replied, assuring her.

'But I want to warn you beforehand. I get bored very easily, so if I don't like it I won't continue,' she added, a smile playing on her face.

This is how my journey with Bebo began; and Bebo's with yoga. We exercised for about a month and then stopped abruptly.

'I think she doesn't like it or may be she just got bored,' I thought to myself, remembering what she had told me during our first meeting.

I had almost forgotten about this episode, when three months later, I received a phone call from Bebo again. By this time I was really intrigued by her.

'Hi Payal, how are you? Can you come to see me? I want to start yoga again,' she said matter-of-factly.

'Yes sure, I will be there,' I replied, thinking she did like it after all.

From that day till now—and it has been almost five years—Bebo has not missed a single session unless she is shooting or is unwell. She lost eight kilos and many inches since we started working out, and looks the best she ever has in her life. But what has been most significant is that her body has undergone a structural change from broad to lean. She has managed to change the shape of her body and achieve what I call the 'perfect ten' by working on her problem areas like the arms, calves, hips, which made her look broad.

Yoga for Bebo has become a way of life that she cannot live without, just as the rest of us cannot live without breathing and eating. There can be no greater pleasure than seeing and feeling the results in your body for yourself. Who doesn't want to fit into their old clothes, not to be conscious of getting photographed, or to eat without feeling guilty? And on top of that have an inner calm that gives your face an unmistakable glow that Bebo has? You can also embrace a brand new perfect ten body. And with it a new way of life: of lifelong health and happiness. It worked for Bebo, and it can for all of you too!

What is a perfect ten?

By now you must be wondering what does perfect ten actually mean? A perfect ten as I call it is the perfect balance of the following ten parameters—height, weight, fat percentage, arms, chest, stomach, waist, hips, thighs, and calves. If you have a proportionate body, that is, the right measurement in all these ten categories, you can be called a perfect ten. This is what gives shape to your body and makes you look sexy. Smita Reddy, a 24-year-old flight attendant was at her ideal body weight of fifty-six kilos as per her 5 feet 5 inches height yet she wondered why she did not look as good as her colleague Manya Patel, who was the same height and weight. The reason is simple. Although Smita's weight was fine yet her body was not well proportioned. Her arms and upper body were extremely thin whereas her lower body was bulkier. As a result, she did not look as good as compared to her perfect ten colleague, Manya, despite being at the right side of the weighing scale. Working out blindly, without knowing where you need to lay stress on and which areas you need to work on more, can never bring about the desired results. You might achieve your ideal body weight like that but you cannot look your best.

Bebo always needs to pay extra attention to her calves and arms as these are her weak areas, and she's prone to put on weight there first.

Gift yourself a measuring tape

Before you start losing weight, the first thing you should do is gift yourself a measuring tape. It is an excellent way to do a regular reality check. Measure yourself from time to time, and focus on your weak areas. You don't need anybody else for this. You can do it all by yourself!

Let us look at the table below. I have illustrated what I mean by perfect ten by taking my own example. As we have already discussed, it takes into consideration ten different attributes of the body—height, weight, fat percentage, arms, chest, stomach, waist, hips, thighs, calves.

Table 2.1: For perfect ten

Attributes of perfect ten	Ideal	Real
Height	5'4"	5'4"
Weight	56–60 kilos	59–60 kilos
Fat percentage	22–24%	24–25%
Arms	10–12 inches	11 inches
Chest	34–36 inches	36 inches
Stomach 4" above naval	26–28 inches	29 inches
Stomach 4" below naval	30–32 inches	33 inches
Waist	26–28 inches	28 inches
Hips	36–38 inches	38 inches
Thighs	19–21 inches	22 inches
Calves	10–12 inches	12 inches

Here I have compared my ideal perfect ten measurements with the real or existing ones. Although I have based this table on myself, you can also measure yourself to find out how many kilos or inches you need to lose and in what area to score a perfect ten. The measurements however can vary as per your age, height and body frame, which can be small, medium, or large.

Although the calculation of a perfect ten will be different for every woman as it depends on your age, height, and body shape, I am using a simpler and broader way to find out whether you are a perfect ten or not. To be a perfect ten, there should be a difference of around 8 inches between your chest and your waist as well as your waist and hip measurements. Also, the size of your chest and your hip should be the same.

I would like to illustrate my point with the help of an example. Let us take three women (W1, W2, W3) who are twenty, thirty, and forty years respectively. The perfect ten figure for all three will be as follows:

W1

Chest: 32–34 inches
Waist: 24–26 inches
Hip: 32–34 inches

W2

Chest: 34–36 inches
Waist: 26–28 inches
Hip. 34–36 inches

W3

Chest: 34–36 inches
Waist: 26–28 inches
Hip: 34–36 inches

This is a way to find out approximately whether you are a perfect ten or not. Looking at the above example, you must have already guessed whether you are a perfect ten or not. If your chest and hip measurements match but the waist does not, you cannot be called a perfect ten. A perfect ten has the perfect curves. All the shapes that we are going to talk about in this chapter lack in one category if not all.

How to get to a perfect ten?

Exercise is the most important aspect of getting to a perfect ten size. Remember, with a diet, you can only lose weight but you can never get a bikini body. And we have already talked about the basic precautions that you need to take in terms of your diet in chapter one. When your body loses fat, it sags down, and you need to exercise to tone it. If you don't, you might just end up looking like a shrivelled raisin. But if you exercise regularly, you can be body beautiful throughout your life.

A case in point is my husband Manish, who drinks two bottles of beer and smokes around ten cigarettes a day. Yet, he is one of the fittest people I know, with a perfect ten body. Manish is a Bollywood yoga expert like me, and he is able to maintain his body even with his so called 'unhealthy habits', only with regular exercise. This chapter is not about losing weight. In this chapter we will talk about getting to the next level, the perfect ten, by changing the shape of your body. What you need to do at this point is to maintain your healthy diet and concentrate on getting a proportionate and toned body, which only exercise can give you. No amount of diet can give you an enviable perfect ten body. So if you want to be able to wear whatever you like and show off a fit and firm body you need to get your act together.

What shape are you?

All of us are born with different body shapes. Damini Goyal, an 18-year-old aspiring model, had broad shoulders and hips but an extremely narrow waist since as long as she could remember. No matter how careless she was, she would never put on weight on her waist. This really amused her and she would love to wear stylish belts to flaunt her middle. This is because Damini has an hour-glass-shaped body.

So let's start by discussing the various body shapes. The most common body shapes found in India are apple, pear, and wine glass. I have two more shapes that I encounter on a regular basis. These are ball and cylinder. In this section, I will talk about each body shape one by one and share with you the specific exercises that you can do for your vulnerable areas. If you practise these exercise regimes regularly, you will be able to change the natural shape of your body. What does this mean? Let me take my own example. I have an apple shaped body, with a tendency to put on weight on my middle. However, since I know this, I have been doing exercises to keep my tummy tucked in. So although my natural body shape is apple, I don't really look like that anymore. With regular and focused exercise, I have been able to achieve the perfect ten body.

The exercises in chapter one help you to lose weight and to get to your ideal body weight. In this chapter, we will go a step ahead. Our goal now is to maintain our weight and change the shape of our body. For instance, an apple-shaped person has to workout focusing on the stomach area, and I have designed this workout keeping this in mind. The same is true for a pear or a wine glass shape. After you have identified your body shape, and thus your weak areas, you too can follow the exercise routine best suited for you to change the shape of your body. This routine will not only help you maintain your weight but also help you become a perfect ten.

Apple

Do you remember how Mala Sinha or Vyjantimala looked in their films? They are both apple-shaped, where the shoulders are broad, middle is heavy, and the legs are comparatively thin. It is almost like an inverted triangle, and fat gets most commonly deposited on the stomach, chest and face. Now you know why sarees suit them better as it does not highlight their middle.

This shape is common in both women and in men. In India, it is often seen that men, after they cross thirty develop a big paunch while the rest of their body is still slim. They all fall under the apple shape. The weak spot for apple-shaped people is the stomach and the surrounding areas. If you are apple-shaped, you don't need to exercise everyday, as the abdominal rectum muscles need to be rested the day after you exercise. So basically you just need to exercise three days in a week. However, on the other days you can do your regular workout, breathing exercises, or any other cardio vascular exercises that you have been doing. All variations of Naukasana or the boat pose are useful for apple-shaped people.

Basic precautions:

1. Never workout on a heavy stomach.
2. Exercise, preferably, two hours after your breakfast and four hours after your lunch.
3. Drink at least 4 to 5 litres of water in a day to avoid constipation and indigestion.
4. There should be a break of at least 10 seconds between each asana in the sequence.
5. If you have any kind of ailments or health related issues

please consult your doctor before doing any exercise or do it under the guidance of a yoga teacher.

6.   Pregnant women should not do these sets of asanas. Also, people with chronic back pain, heart related problems, and hernia should avoid these asanas.

Where: Choose a place which has fresh air circulation preferably a garden, a terrace, or a workout place in your house.

What you need: A yoga mat, a bottle of water, and a hand or face towel. You can also play some nice slow music in the background if you like.

Warming up: Spread the mat on the floor and sit in a comfortable position. Take five to ten long breaths to relax yourself, then lie down on your back and stretch yourself by raising your hands up and toes downward about five times:

A.   Now start the series of Naukasana (boat pose)

1.   Ardha Naukasana: lie down on your back with your feet together and your palms resting on your thighs. Inhale slowly and raise one leg, simultaneously raise the upper body and hands upwards, towards the toe. Hold it for 30 seconds while breathing normally, then slowly come down and repeat the same with the other leg.

2.   Ardha Triyak Naukasana: lie down on your back with your feet together and your palms resting on your thighs. Inhale slowly and raise one leg up, then raise the upper body upwards while twisting towards the opposite side. Hold for 30 seconds while breathing normally. Repeat the asana with

the other leg.

3.   Poorna Triyak Naukasana: lie down on your back with your feet together and your palms resting on your thighs. Inhale slowly and raise both legs up then raise the upper body and hands upwards towards the toes. Now turn your full body towards the right side on your hip. Repeat the process with the other side. Hold for 30 seconds on each side.

4.   Naukasana: lie down on your back with your feet together and your palms resting on your thighs. Inhale and raise both legs up, then pull the upper body off the floor. Hold for 30 seconds while breathing normally keeping your hands parallel to the floor. Slowly come back to the starting position.

5.   Naukasana variation 1: lie down on your back, feet together, palms resting on your thighs. Inhale slowly and raise both legs up, folding your arms across your chest. Hold for 30 seconds while breathing normally and slowly come down to the starting position.

6.   Naukasana variation 2: lie down on your back, feet together, palms resting on your thighs slowly inhale and raise both legs up and raising your arms parallel to your ears. Hold for 20 seconds while breathing normally and slowly come down to the starting position.

Repeat these six asanas, 4 sets, relaxing for 2 minutes after each set. Also, don't forget to do the counter pose, on this case, 1 set of Kati Chakrasana. Hold for 20 seconds on each side. These asanas are good for burning fat from your stomach area, and help tone your abdominal muscles. They also improve your digestion or any stomach related problems that you might have. I would recommend this for people with diabetes.

B.   Next, you need to do the Setubandhasana or the bridge pose.

Lie on your back, and bend your knees. Keep your feet close to your hips with hands by the side, palms resting on the floor.

Inhale slowly and raise your back higher as much as you can without any pressure on your neck. Hold for 20 to 30 seconds while breathing normally for 2 sets.

C.   The third kind of exercise for the apple-shaped person is Kriya and Pranayam in sitting position; for example Sukhasana. This helps to cleanse the body and enhance breathing.

1.   Kapalbhati kriya: Exhale forcefully through your nose, 2 strokes in 1 second. If you are a beginner start with 25 strokes (2 rounds) and do it slowly that is, only 1 stroke in 1 second. As you get used to it and can do it with ease, increase up to 50 strokes (4 rounds). Advanced practitioners can do 100 strokes (5 rounds) at a stretch but I would not recommend this for beginners. Heart patients or people with high blood pressure should avoid this kriya. If you do this on a regular basis, it will balance and strengthen the nervous system and tone your digestive organs. It also has a cleansing effect on the lungs and is good for any respiratory problems.

2.   Anulom Vilom: Use the thumb of your right hand

to close your right nostril and inhale from the left nostril, then close your left nostril with your right hand's index and middle fingers and exhale from the right nostril. Now in the reverse manner, inhale with the right nostril, close your right nostril with your right hand thumb, and then exhale with the left. This forms 1 round of Anulom Vilom Pranayam. Do this for 5 rounds. When done on a regular basis, Pranayam purifies 72,000 nerves (nadis) in the body, and in turn balances the body temperature.

Pear

The pears are heavier on the lower half of their body. They tend to put on weight on their hips, thighs, outer thighs, inner thighs, and calves. Asha Parikh and Mumtaz in their time were naturally pear shaped, but with regular exercise they have been able to maintain their figures. A pear-shaped body is most common among women. In such a body type, you need to exercise everyday for about an hour.

Basic precautions:

1. Never workout on a heavy stomach.
2. Exercise preferably two hours after your breakfast and four hours after your lunch.
3. Avoid constipation and indigestion.
4. Drink at least 4 to 5 litres of water in a day.
5. There should be a break of at least 10 seconds between each asana in the sequence.
6. If you have any kind of ailments or health related issues please consult your doctor before doing any exercise, or

do it under the guidance of a yoga teacher.

7. Pregnant women should not do these sets of asanas. Also, people with chronic back pain, heart related problems, and hernia should avoid these asanas.

Where: Choose a place, which has fresh air circulation preferably a garden, a terrace, or a workout place in your house.

What you need: A yoga mat, a bottle of water, and a hand or face towel. You can also play some nice slow music in the background if you like.

Warming up: Spread the mat on the floor and sit in a comfortable position. Take five to ten long breaths to relax yourself, then lie down on your back and stretch yourself by raising your hands upwards and toes downward about 5 times.

1. Utkatasana (chair pose against the wall): Stand at a distance of one and a half feet from the wall. Place your back against the wall and bend your knees at an angle of ninety degrees from the floor. Hold this pose for 30 seconds to 1 minute while breathing normally, repeat in 5 sets. This asana is extremely good for your thigh muscles.

You should not do this asana if you have arthritis. I recommend a different posture for people with arthritis. Sit on the floor while resting your palms on the ground for back support. Now spread your feet apart in the same width as your shoulders. Raise your left leg up, hold it for 10 seconds, then slowly bring it back to the original position. Repeat the process with the other leg, making sure that you breathe normally. Do three sets of this asana.

2. Utkatasana: Face the wall, support your body with your hand and bend your knees at an angle of 90 degrees from the floor. Raise your heels up and hold for 30 seconds, then move your heels up and down 20 to 25 times. This forms one set. Do 3 sets of this asana. This asana is beneficial for your calf muscles as well as your thighs. You should not do this asana if you have arthritis.

3. Cat pose variation: Place your hands under your shoulders. Your knees should be apart in the same level. Now raise your right leg up straight, without applying pressure on your back, and make a major contraction on your butt muscles. Hold this position for 45 seconds and contract your butt 20 to 25 times. Repeat the asana with the other leg three times. This exercise tones your butt muscles.

4. Ek Pada Ardha Halasana variation: Lie down on your back on the floors. Keep your hands straight at shoulder level with the palm resting on the floor. Raise your right leg a ninety degree angle from the floor, then turn it towards the right side of the floor till you feel the contraction in your inner thighs. Hold for 20 seconds, then turn your left till you get the contraction on your outer thighs. Hold for 20 seconds, then keep changing the leg position in the same way 20 to 30 times. Repeat the entire process with the other leg three times. This asana is useful for your inner as well as outer thigh.

5. Dhanurasana: Lie down on the floor on your stomach. Bend your knees, hold your ankles with your hands and inhale. Now raise your upper body and pull your legs up as well. Hold for 15 to 20 seconds. Repeat twice. This

asana works on your leg muscles, stomach, and back.

6. Gomukhasana: Sit on the floor stretching your legs forward. Bend both your knees slightly. Place your left leg under your right thigh, and take your right leg over your left leg making sure one knee is under the other. Now take your right hand behind your back with your palm facing downwards, and place your left hand behind. Try holding both your palms together, making sure your entire back is straight and aligned with your neck. Breathe normally once you are in this posture. Repeat the same with the other leg and hand positions. Hold each side for 30 seconds twice.

7. Ek Padasana: This asana is done in a standing position. Place your feet together and raise your hands up in Namaskar position. Now bend forward and simultaneously raise your right leg up straight, making your posture in T shape. Hold for 30 seconds on each leg. Repeat it 3 times.

8. Garudasana: This asana is also done in standing position. Bend your knees slightly, and entangle your right leg on to the left calf. Similarly, entangle your right hand on to your left hand and bring it to the chest level. Hold it there, breathing normally for 20 seconds. Follow the same with the other leg and hand. Repeat twice.

These sets of asanas are good for building strength and toning the muscles of the legs and the hips. People with chronic knee problems and arthritis should not do these asanas.

9. The last kind of exercise for the pear-shaped person is Pranayam in sitting position.

Anulom Vilom: Use your right hand to close your right nostril and inhale from the left nostril, then close your left nostril with your right hand's index and middle fingers and exhale from the right nostril. Now reverse the hands and fingers to inhale with the right nostril and exhale with the left. This forms 1 round of Anulom Vilom Pranayam. Do this for 5 rounds.

How Kareena became a perfect ten

In Bebo's case, I made her do exercises that work on weak areas, and her body has responded excellently. Although Kareena is pear shaped, her butt is her asset. Her arms were heavy and her shoulders were broad. Hence, Suryanamaskars worked wonders for her to get her upper body into shape. Some other upper body exercises; like holding Parvatasana for a minute, push ups, and holding the postures for longer have also helped her to get the lean look that she sports today.

Bebo also had heavy calves, and for that I made her stand near a wall, with her back facing the wall and then made her bend in a chair position for more than a minute. This was followed by raising her heels up and balancing the body on her toes. I made her hold her position for more than a minute. Bebo's lower body is her strength and she can do as much exercise as she wants with her lower body. But her upper body and core are weak, and to strengthen these I made her do Naukasana variations. I also made her do Simhasana (lion pose) for high cheekbones and helped make her cheeks thinner by sucking it inwards, and holding it there. Yes, you can even change the shape of your face with yoga! But these are only a few of the exercises that we did.

The twelve asanas forming one round of Suryanamaskar

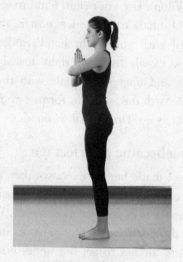

Namaskar Mudra

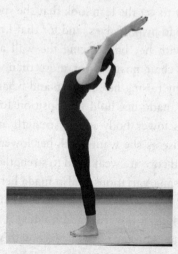

Back bending Chakrasana

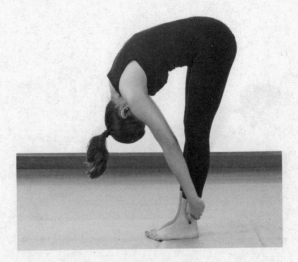

Padahastasana

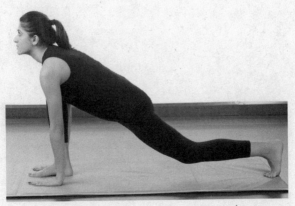

Ashwa Sanchalanasana with right leg forward

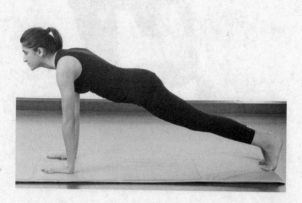

Santolanasana

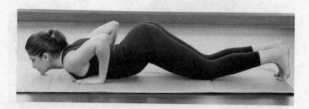

Shashtanga Mudra

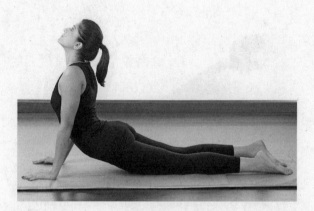

Sarpasana

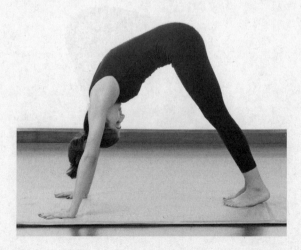

Parvatasana

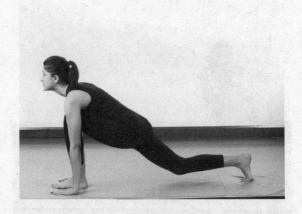

Ashwa Sanchalanasana with left leg forward

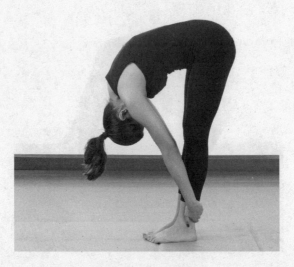

Padahastasana

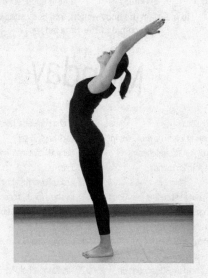

Back bending Chakrasana

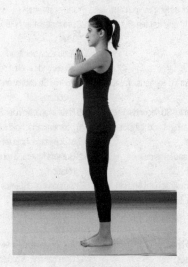

Namaskar Mudra

Bebo's exercise routine

Age: **30**   Weight: **54 kilos**   Sessions: **1 hour each, six days a week**
Target: **To maintain the body weight, and body shape as well
as becoming fitter than before.**

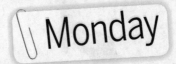

Monday

Warm up exercises:

1   5 to 6 minutes of warm up exercises in
    the form of dynamic stretches
2   Suryanamaskar: 25 rounds

Full body work out in standing positions:

3   Side bending Chakrasana: hold for 30
    seconds on each side, 1 set
4   Ardha Chandrasana: hold for 30
    seconds on each side, 1 set
5   Trikonasana: hold for 30 seconds on
    each side, 1 set
6   Pada Hastasana: hold for 30 seconds
    (you can hold it for as long as you can)
7   Vrikshasana: right and left leg, 30
    seconds

Sitting positions:

8   Ustrasana: hold for 20 seconds on each
    side, 1 set
9   Bhadrasana: hold for 30 seconds, 1 set
10 Janu Shirshasana: right and left side:
    30 seconds, 1 set
11 Vakrasana: right and left side:
    30 seconds, 1 set
12 Ardha Matsyendrasana: right and left
    side: 30 seconds, 1 set

Supine positions:

13 Shavasana: deep breathing (slow and
    rhythmic 2 minutes)
14 Supta Tadasana: hold for 10 seconds,
    1 set

15 Ardha Halasana: hold for 20 seconds on
    each angle, 1 set
16 Saral Matsyasana: hold for 20 seconds,
    1 set
17 Ardha Pavanmuktasana: right and left
    leg, hold for 30 seconds, 1 set
18 Pavanmuktasana: hold for 30 seconds,
    1 set
19 Setubandhasana: hold for 20 seconds,
    1 set
20 Naukasana: hold for 30 seconds, 3 sets
21 Vipreetkarni: hold for 30 seconds, 1 set

Prone positions:

22 Bhujangasana: hold for 30 seconds,
    1 set
23 Ardha Shalabhasana: right and left leg,
    30 seconds each, 1 set
24 Poorna Shalabhasana: hold for 30
    seconds, 1 set
25 Naukasana: hold for 20 seconds, 1 set
26 Dhanurasana: hold for 30 seconds, 1 set
27 Makarasana: hold for 1 minute
28 Brahma Mudra: 3 rounds (neck
    rotation)
29 Simhasana: 3 rounds (20 seconds
    each)
30 Kapalbhati: 100 to 250 strokes (2 to 4
    rounds)
31 Anulom Vilom Pranayam: 10 rounds
32 Om chanting: 5 rounds with relaxation

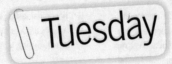

> To me the only way to stay fit is through yoga and that's the way I would advise my fans to live their lives!

Tuesday

Warm up for 5-6 minutes through static or dynamic stretches

1 Suryanamaskar: 30 to 40 rounds
2 Utkatasana: hold for 30 seconds, 1 set movement for 30 seconds hold for 10 seconds
3 Ardha Chandrasana: hold on each side for 30 seconds
4 Tadasana: hold for 30 seconds, 2 sets
5 Uttanasana: hold for 30 seconds, 3 sets
6 Garudasana: hold for 20 seconds on each leg.
7 Ek Pada Uttan Angusthasana (leg to the side): hold for 30 seconds on each leg
8 Natrajasana: hold for 30 seconds on each leg

Sitting positions:
9 Ardha Matsyendrasana: right and left hold for 30 seconds each
10 Paschimottanasana: hold for 20 to 30 seconds
11 Akarna Dhanurasana: right and left: hold for 30 seconds each
12 Ustrasana: hold for 30 seconds
13 Sharnagat Mudra: forward bend, hold

for 20 seconds
14 Ugrasana: hold for 30 seconds
15 Padmasana: hold for 30 seconds
16 Supta Vagrasana: hold for 30 seconds
17 Kapotasana: hold for 30 seconds

Supine positions:
18 Shavasana: 2 minutes
19 Sarvanganasa: hold for 30 seconds
20 Matsyasana: hold for 30 seconds
21 Halasana: hold for 30 seconds
22 Setubandhasana: hold for 30 seconds

Prone positions:
23 Bhujangasana: hold for 30 seconds
24 Poorna Shalabhasana: hold for 30 seconds
25 Naukasana: hold for 30 seconds
26 Dhanurasana: hold for 30 seconds
27 Brahma Mudra: 2 to 4 rounds
28 Simhasana: 5 to 10 rounds
29 Kapalbhati: 120 strokes, 5 rounds
30 Bhastrika: 3 to 5 rounds
31 Anulom Vilom: 12 rounds
32 Bhramari: 12 rounds
33 Om chanting: 5 rounds with relaxation

Wednesday

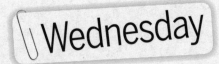

Wednesday is the day for a complete cardio workout. The sequence is very important in this workout and is a mix of sitting, standing supine and prone positions.

1 spot jogging: 30 seconds
2 Jumping jack: 30 seconds
3 Side twist: 30 seconds
4 Suryanamaskar: 10 rounds
5 Kapalbhati: 100 strokes
6 Spot jogging: 30 seconds
7 Jumping jack: 30 seconds
8 Side twist: 30 seconds
9 Chandranamaskar: 10 rounds
10 Kapalbhati: 100 strokes
11 Repeat spot jogging, jumping jack, side twist
12 Suryanamaskar: 10 rounds
13 Kapalbhati: 100 strokes
14 Repeat jogging, jumping jack and side twist
15 Chandranamaskar: 10 rounds
16 Kapalbhati: 100 strokes
17 Repeat: jogging, jumping jack, and side twist
18 Suryanamaskar: 10 rounds
19 Kapalbhati: 100 rounds
20 Repeat jogging, jumping jack, and side twist
21 Chandranamaskar: 10 rounds
22 Kapalbhati: 100 strokes
23 Shavasana: 5 minutes
24 Crocodile pose variations 1, 2, 3, 4, 5 and 6 (spinal twist)
25 Pavanmuktasana: 20 seconds
26 Dhanurasana: 30 seconds
27 Naukasana: 30 seconds
28 Brahma Mudra: 2 to 4 rounds
29 Bhramari Pranayam: 12 rounds
30 Om chanting: 5 rounds with relaxation

Thursday

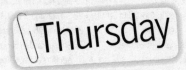

Stretching

On Thursdays we only do stretches and no Suryanamaskars due to a hectic workout the previous day.

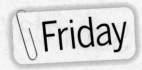

Friday

Warm up exercises

1 5 to 6 minutes of warm up exercises in the form of dynamic or static stretches
2 Suryanamaskar: 25 rounds
3 Santolanasana: hold for 15 seconds, movement for 15 seconds, hold for 10 seconds
4 Santolanasana variation 1: hold for 30 seconds, right and left arms
5 Santolanasana variation 2: hold for 15 seconds, right and left arms up, sideways
6 Santolanasana variation 3: hold for 15 seconds with one arm back, each side
7 Ek Pada Hasta Santolanasana: hold for 15 seconds, right and left sides
8 Ek Padasana: hold for 30 seconds each, right and left
9 Natrajasana: hold for 30 seconds each, right and left

10 Setubandhasana: hold for 30 seconds
11 Setubandhasana variation 1 with straight legs: hold for 15 seconds
12 Trikonasana: hold for 30 seconds
13 Parighasana: hold for 30 seconds, right and left side

Sitting positions:
14 Ardha Matsyendrasana: 30 seconds, right and left side

Prone positions:
15 Bhujangasana: 10 seconds, 2 sets
16 Sarpasana: 10 seconds, 2 sets
17 Dhanurasana: 10 seconds, 2 sets
18 Shavasana: 2 minutes
19 Kapalbhati: 120 strokes, 5 rounds

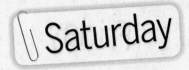

Saturday

On Saturdays we mainly do balancing and inverted postures.
Start with a warm up of 5 to 6 minutes Suryanamaskar and Chandranamaskar: 15 rounds each

Standing and balancing positions:
1 Vrikshasana: hold for 30 seconds on each leg
2 Garudasana: hold for 30 seconds on each leg
3 Natrajasana: hold for 30 seconds on each leg
4 Ek Padasana: hold for 30 seconds on each leg
5 Ardha Baddha Padmottanasana: hold for 30 seconds on each leg

Sitting positions:
6 Merudandasana: hold for 30 seconds
7 Naukasana: hold for 30 seconds to 60 seconds, 2 sets

8 Naukasana variation 1: hold for 30 seconds, 2 sets
9 Naukasana variation 2: hold for 30 seconds, 2 sets

Supine positions:
10 Vipreetkarni: hold for 30 seconds
11 Sarvanganasa: hold for 30 seconds
12 Poorna Halasana: hold for 30 seconds
13 Matsyasana: hold for 20 seconds

Prone positions:
14 Bhujangasana: hold for 30 seconds
15 Dhanurasana: hold for 30 seconds
16 Sarpasana: hold for 30 seconds
17 Brahma Mudra: 2 to 3 rounds
18 Kapalbhati: 120 strokes, 3 rounds
19 Anulom Vilom: 12 rounds
20 Om chanting: 5 rounds
21 Shavasana: 2 minutes

Bebo does not have a weight problem any longer. She's been at her ideal body weight for sometime now and our aim is to maintain her perfect ten figure.

Wine glass

If you have a wine glass shaped body, your upper body will be significantly heavier in comparison to your middle or lower body. A wine glass person has usually very skinny legs. Moushami Chatterjee has the quintessential wine glass physique. This again is more common among women with a tendency to put on weight on their hands, chest, upper back, and shoulders.

Basic precautions:

1. Never workout on a heavy stomach.
2. Exercise preferably 2 hours after your breakfast and 4 hours after your lunch.
3. Drink at least 4 to 5 litres of water in a day to avoid constipation and indigestion.
4. There should be a break of at least 10 seconds between each asana in the sequence.
5. If you have any kind of ailments or health related issues, please consult your doctor before doing any exercise, or do it under the guidance of a yoga teacher.
6. Pregnant women should not do these sets of asanas. Also, people with chronic back pain, heart related problems, and hernia should avoid these asanas.

Where: Choose a place which has fresh air circulation preferably a garden, a terrace, or a workout place in your house.

What you need: A yoga mat, a bottle of water, and a hand or face towel. You can also play some nice slow music in the background if you like.

Warming up: Spread the mat on the floor and sit in a comfortable position. Take five to ten long breaths to relax yourself, then lie down on your back and stretch yourself by raising your hands upwards and toes downward about five times.

1. Suryanamaskar: Start with at least 15 to 20 rounds of the series of 12 postures.

2. Ek Padasana in standing position: Place your legs and your palms together. Interlock your fingers with each other, inhale and raise your hands upwards to stretch as much as you can. Now exhale slowly while bending forward and down with your right leg up. Make sure that your right leg, back, and your hands are in a straight line while making a 90-degree angle from the floor. Repeat the process with the other leg. Hold for 20 seconds; each leg for 3 sets.

3. Ek Padasana variation in standing position: Place your legs together and your hands by the side. Slowly take your hands to your back from the sides, interlocking your fingers with each other and fixing your palms and inhale. Stretch your hands behind, bend your upper body forward while raising your right leg up. Make a 90-degree angle from the floor. Do the same with the other leg. Hold for 20 seconds for each leg; 3 sets.

4. Santolanasana in sitting position: Sit in cat pose straighten your knees, move the shoulders forward, and push the buttock downwards until the body is

straight like position no. 5 of Suryanamaskar. Hold for 30 seconds; 3 times.

5. Santolanasana variation 1: same as Santolanasana with bent elbows, close to your body. Hold for 30 seconds for 3 sets.

6. Santolanasana variation 2: Sit in cat pose, straighten your knees, move the shoulders forward, and push the buttock downwards until the body is parallel to the floor. Slowly turn your full body to the right side and raise your left hand up to your shoulder's level. Make sure your upper body weight is on your right hand and lower body weight on your left leg. Repeat the same with the other side. Hold 20 seconds for 3 sets.

These asanas are good for toning and strengthening your upper body especially the arms, shoulders, and chest muscles.

Relax in Shavasana for 5 minutes.

7. The last kind of breathing exercise for the pear-shaped person is Pranayam in sitting position (Sukhasana).

Anulom Vilom: Use the thumb of your right hand to close your right nostril and inhale from the left nostril, then close your left nostril with your right hand's index and middle fingers and exhale from the right nostril. Now in the reverse manner inhale with the right nostril, close your right nostril with your right hand thumb then exhale with the left. This forms 1 round of Anulom Vilom Pranayam. Do this for 5 rounds. When done on a regular basis, this Pranayam purifies 72,000 nerves (nadis) in the body, and in turn balances the body temperature.

8. Om chanting for 5 minutes.

Cylinder

A person with a cylinder-shaped body may not necessarily be fat, but has no curves in their body. Minakshi Sheshadree can fall under this category. This is especially a problem in some women who don't have curves in the waist, hips, and stomach line. For a cylinder body shape, you need to walk three days a week and workout on the other three days. The seventh day is for relaxation of the muscles.

Basic precautions:

1. Never workout on a heavy stomach
2. Exercise preferably 2 hours after your breakfast and 4 hours after your lunch.
3. Drink at least 4 to 5 litres of water in a day to avoid constipation and indigestion.
4. There should be a break of at least 10 seconds between each asana in the sequence.
5. If you have any kind of ailments or health related issues, please consult your doctor before doing any exercise, or do it under the guidance of a yoga teacher.
6. Pregnant women should not do these set of asanas. Also, people with chronic back pain, heart related problems, and hernia should avoid these asanas.

Where: Choose a place which has fresh air circulation preferably a garden, a terrace, or a workout place in your house.
What you need: A yoga mat, a bottle of water, and a hand or face towel. You can also play some nice slow music in the background if you like.
Warming up: Spread the mat on the floor and sit in a comfortable

position. Take 5 to 10 long breaths to relax yourself, then lie down on your back and stretch yourself by raising your hands upwards and toes downward about 5 times.

1. Suryanamaskar: 10 rounds, normally.
2. Suryanamaskar: 10 rounds with sit-ups. Do 5 sit-ups, then 1 Suryanamaskar. Repeat this for 10 rounds.

Remember to relax for 2 minutes after each set. Also, don't forget to do the counter pose (Kati Chakrasana) after each asana.

3. Ardha Chandrasana: standing positions, feet together, hands by the side, put your right leg forward, bend your right knee at an angle of 90 degrees to the floor push your left leg behind till you feel the stretch on your left thigh, then inhale and raise your hands up in Namaskar Mudra with straightened elbows and arched back. Hold for 30 seconds with normal breathing. Repeat with the other leg for 3 sets each. This asana tones your thighs, butt, and your arms and it stretches your abdominal and back muscles.

4. Naukasana: Inhale and raise both legs up, then raise the upper body off the floor. Hold for 30 seconds while breathing normally. Repeat it for 5 sets. This asana tones your abdominal muscles, improves digestion and is good for diabetes.

5. Side bending Chakrasana: While standing, put your feet together with your hands on the sides. Now raise your right hand up and stretch while bending your body towards the left side. Hold for 30 seconds, then come back to the original position. Repeat it with the other side for 5 sets. This asana is beneficial for

reducing fat from your love handles and arms, and is also good for patients of asthma. It is good for your side muscles.

6.   Dhanurasana on the stomach: Lie down on the floor on your stomach. Bend your knees, hold your ankles with your hands, and inhale while raising your upper body and your legs up slowly. Hold up to 15 to 20 seconds. Repeat it for 2 sets. This asana stretches your leg muscles, stomach, and back. If you have a severe back pain, please avoid this asana.

7.   Next do Pranayam and kriyas in sitting position.

   • Kapalbhati kriya: Exhale forcefully through your nose, 2 strokes in 1 second. Do 500 strokes at a stretch. This is not recommended for heart patients or people with high blood pressure.

   • Anulom Vilom: Use the thumb of your right hand to close your right nostril and inhale from the left nostril, then close your left nostril with your right hand's index and middle fingers and exhale from the right nostril. Now in the reverse manner inhale with the right nostril, close your right nostril with your right hand's thumb then exhale with the left. This forms 1 round of Anulom Vilom Pranayam. Do this for 5 rounds. When done on a regular basis, this Pranayam purifies 72,000 nerves (nadis) in the body, and in turn balances the body temperature.

   • Suryabhedan: Inhale from the right nostril and exhale from the left. Repeat it 10 to 15 rounds.

Ball

A ball-shaped person is overall round in appearance. This reminds me instantly of Guddi Maruti. If you fall in this category, you would need to workout everyday.

Basic precautions:

1. Never workout on a heavy stomach.
2. Exercise preferably 2 hours after your breakfast and 4 hours after your lunch.
3. Drink at least 4 to 5 litres of water in a day to avoid constipation and indigestion.
4. There should be a break of at least 10 seconds between each asana in the sequence.

Where: Choose a place which has fresh air circulation preferably a garden, a terrace, or a workout place in your house.

What you need: A yoga mat, a bottle of water, and a hand or face towel. You can also play some nice slow music in the background if you like.

Warming up: Spread the mat on the floor and sit in a comfortable position. Take 5 to 10 long breaths to relax yourself, then lie down on your back and stretch yourself by raising your hands upwards and toes downwards about 5 times.

1. Begin with cardiovascular exercises for 30 to 40 minutes, then relax for 10 minutes.
2. Suryanamaskar: 30 to 40 times with breaks. First start with only 10 rounds, then gradually increase it to 30 in a month.

   People with this body shape can do all asanas meant for apple, pear, wine, and cylinder shapes.

3. Ardha Naukasana: Inhale and raise one leg up, then pull your upper body upwards. Hold it for 30 seconds while breathing normally. Repeat the asana with the other leg.

4. Triyak Naukasana: Inhale and raise one leg up, then pull the upper body upwards while twisting it. Hold for 30 seconds while breathing normally. Repeat the asana with the other leg.

5. Naukasana: Inhale and raise both legs up, then pull your upper body off the floor. Hold for 30 seconds while breathing normally.

    Repeat these three asanas four times, relaxing for 2 minutes after each round. Also, don't forget to do the counter pose after each asana.

6. Next, you need to do the Setubandhasana or the bridge pose. Lie on your back, and bend your knees. Keep your feet close to your hips with hands by the side, and palms resting on the floor. Inhale slowly and raise your back as high as you can without any pressure on your back. Hold for 20 to 30 seconds while breathing normally.

7. Chair pose against the wall: stand at a distance of two feet from the wall. Place your back against the wall and bend your knees at a 90 degrees angle from the floor. Hold this pose for 30 seconds to 1 minute while breathing normally. Repeat five times. This asana is extremely good for your thigh muscles. You should not do this asana if you have arthritis.

8. Utkatasana: Now turn the other way round and face the wall. Take the wall's support with your hand and bend your knees at 90 degree to the floor. Raise your heels up

and hold for 30 seconds, then move your heels up and down 20 to 25 times. This forms one set. Repeat this thrice. This asana is beneficial for your calf muscles as well as your thighs. You should not do this asana if you have arthritis.

9. The cat pose: Sit on the floor with palms resting on the floor like a cat. Place your hands under your shoulder level. Your knees should be apart in same level. Now raise your right leg up straight, without applying pressure on your back, make a major contraction on your butt muscles. Hold this position for 45 seconds and contract your butt 20 to 25 times. Repeat the asana with the other leg three times. This exercise is good for your butt muscles.

10. In the same position, place your arms apart with palms facing outside and repeat the same procedure.

11. In the same position, place your arms apart with palms facing inside at the chest level and repeat the same procedure. This will helps you to reduce the fat from your arms and back.

12. Next do Pranayam and kriya in sitting position. Kapalbhati kriya: Exhale forcefully through your nose, two strokes in 1 second. Do 25 strokes at a stretch. This is not recommended for heart patients or people with high blood pressure.

13. Anulom Vilom: Use the thumb of your right hand to close your right nostril and inhale from the left nostril, then close your left nostril with your right hand's index and middle fingers and exhale from the right nostril. Now in the reverse manner inhale with the right nostril, close your right nostril with your right hand thumb then

exhale with the left. This forms 1 round of Anulom Vilom Pranayam. Do this for 5 rounds. When done on a regular basis, this Pranayam purifies 72,000 nerves (nadis) in the body, and in turn balances the body temperature. This forms 1 round of Bhastrika. Repeat 4 rounds.

14. Ardha Naukasana: Lie down on your back with your feet together and your palms resting on your thighs. Inhale slowly and raise one leg up, simultaneously raise your upper body and hands upwards, towards the toe. Hold for 30 seconds while breathing normally. Repeat. Slowly come down and with the other leg.

15. Ardha Triyak Naukasana: Lie down on your back with your feet together and your palms resting on your thighs. Inhale slowly and raise one leg up, then raise your upper body upwards while twisting towards the opposite side Hold for 30 seconds while breathing normally. Slowly come down and repeat the same with the other leg.

16. Poorna Triyak Naukasana: Lie down on your back with your feet together and your palms resting on your thighs. Inhale slowly and raise both legs up. Then raise your upper body and hands upwards towards your toes. Now turn your full body towards the right side of your right hip. Repeat with the other side. Hold for 30 seconds on each side.

17. Naukasana: Lie down on your back with your feet together and your palms resting on your thighs. Inhale and raise both legs up, then raise upper body off the floor. Hold for 30 seconds while breathing normally keeping your hands parallel to the floor. Slowly come back to the starting position.

18. Naukasana variation 1: Lie down on your back, feet together, palms resting on your thighs. Inhale slowly and raise both legs up, folding your arms across your chest. Hold for 30 seconds while breathing normally and slowly come down to the starting position.

19. Naukasana variation 2: Lie down on your back, feet together, palms resting on your thighs. Inhale slowly and raise both legs up, raising your arms parallel to your ears. Hold for 20 seconds while breathing normally and slowly come down to the starting position.

Repeat these 6 asanas, 4 sets, relaxing for 2 minutes after each set. Also, don't forget to do the counter pose (Kati Chakrasana; hold for 20 seconds, each side 1 set) after each asana. These asanas are good for burning fat from your stomach area, and help tone your abdominal muscles. They also improve your digestion, or any stomach related problems that you might have. I would recommend this for people having diabetes.

20. Next, you need to do the Setubandhasana or the bridge pose.

a) Lie on your back, and bend your knees. Keep your feet close to your hips with hands by the side, and palms resting on the floor. Inhale slowly and raise your back as high as you can without any pressure on your neck. Hold for 20 to 30 seconds while breathing normally for 2 sets. The third kind of cleaning and breathing exercise for the ball-shaped person is kriya and Pranayam in sitting position (Sukhasana).

b) Kapalbhati kriya (active exhalation): Exhale

forcefully through your nose, two strokes in 1 second. If you are a beginner, start with 25 strokes (2 rounds) and do it slowly (1 stroke in 1 second). As you get used to it and can do it with ease, increase it to 50 strokes (4 rounds). Advanced practitioners can do 100 strokes (5 rounds) at a stretch but I would not recommend this for beginners. Heart patients or people with high blood pressure, should avoid this kriya. If you do this on a regular basis, it will balance and strengthen the nervous system and tone your digestive organs. It also has a cleansing effect on the lungs and is good for any respiratory related problems.

c)   Anulom Vilom: Use the thumb of your right hand to close your right nostril and inhale from the left nostril, then close your left nostril with your right hand's index and middle fingers and exhale from the right nostril. Now in the reverse manner inhale with the right nostril, close your right nostril with your right hand thumb then exhale with the left. This forms 1 round of Anulom Vilom Pranayam. Do this for 5 rounds. When done on a regular basis, this Pranayam purifies 72, 000 nerves (nadis) in the body, and in turn balances the body temperature.

21.   Chair pose against the wall: Stand at a distance of 1½ feet from the wall. Place your back against the wall and bend your knees at a 90-degrees angle to the floor. Hold this pose for 30 seconds to 1 minute while breathing normally. Do 5 sets. This asana is extremely good for your thigh muscles.

You should not do this asana if you have arthritis. I recommend a different posture for people with arthritis. Sit on the floor and spread your feet shoulder width apart, palms resting on the floor for back support. Raise your left leg up, hold for 10 seconds, then slowly bring it back to the original position. Repeat the process with the other leg, making sure that you breathe normally. Repeat 3 sets.

22. Utkatasana: Now turn the other way round and facing the wall, support yourself against the wall with your hands and bend your knees at 90 degrees from the floor. Raise your heels up and hold for 30 seconds, then move your heels up and down 20 to 25 times. This forms one set. Do 3 sets. This asana is beneficial for your calf muscles as well as your thighs.

    You should not do this asana if you have arthritis.

23. Ek Pada Vyaghrasana variation: Sit on the floor with palm resting on the floor like a cat. Place your hands under your shoulders. Your knees should be apart in the same level. Now raise your right leg up straight, without applying pressure on your back, and make major contraction in your butt muscles. Hold this position for 25 seconds. Move your leg up and down and contracting your butt muscles 20 to 25 times. Repeat with the other leg. Do 3 sets each. This exercise is good for your butt muscles.

24. Ek Pada Ardha Halasana: Lie down on your back on the floor. Keep your hands straight at shoulder level with the palms resting on the floor. Raise your right leg at a 90-degree angle to the floor, then turn your leg towards

the right side till you feel the contraction in your inner thighs. Hold for 20 seconds, then turn towards the left side of the floor till you get a contraction in your outer thighs. Hold for 20 seconds, then keep changing the leg position in the same way 20 to 30 times. Repeat with the other leg. Do 3 sets each. This asana is useful for your inner, as well as, outer thighs.

25. Dhanurasana: Lie down on your stomach on the floor. Bend your knees, hold your ankles with your hands while inhaling. Raise your upper body and raise your legs up as well. Hold for up to 15 to 20 seconds. Repeat it for 2 sets. This asana tones your arms, legs, stomach, and back muscles.

26. Gomukhasana: Sit on the floor stretching your legs forward. Slightly bend both your knees. Place your left leg under your right thigh, and take your right leg over your left leg making sure one knee is under the other. Now take your right hand behind your back with your palm facing downwards, and place your left hand behind your right hand. Try holding both your palms together, making sure your entire back is straight and aligned with your neck. Breathe normally once you are in this posture. Repeat with the other leg and hand positions. Hold each side for 30 seconds do this for 3 sets. This asana strengthens and tones your arms, legs, and back.

27. Ek Padasana: This asana is done in a standing position. Place your feet together and raise your hands up in Namaskar position. Now bend forward and simultaneously raise your right leg up straight, making

your posture in a T shape. Hold for 30 seconds on each leg. Repeat for 3 sets each. This asana also strengthens and tones your arms, legs, and back. It also helps in achieving a balance between the body and the mind.

28. Garudasana: This asana is also done in a standing position. Bend your knees slightly, and entangle your right leg on to the left calf. Similarly, entangle your right hand on to your left hand and bring it to the chest level. Hold it there, breathing normally for 20 seconds. Follow the same with the other leg and hand. Repeat it for 2 sets each.

29. Suryanamaskar: Start with at least 15 to 20 rounds of the series of 12 postures.

30. Ek Padasana (in standing position): Place your legs and your palms together. Interlock your fingers with each other, inhale, and raise your hands upwards to stretch as much as you can. Now slowly exhale while bending forward and down with your right leg up. Make sure that your right leg, back and your hands are in a straight line while making a 90-degree angle to the floor. Repeat the process with the other leg. Hold for 20 seconds and repeat with each leg for 3 sets.

31. Ek Padasana (variation) in standing position: Place your legs together and your hands by the side. Slowly take your hands to your back from the sides, interlocking your fingers with each other. Fix your palms and inhale. Stretch your hands behind while bending your upper body forward and raising your right leg up to make a 90-degree angle from the floor. Repeat the same with the other leg. Hold for 20 seconds and repeat with each leg for 3 sets.

32. Santolanasana in sitting position: Sit in cat pose, straighten your knees, move the shoulders forward, and press the buttock downwards until the body is straight like position no. 5 of Suryanamaskar. Hold for 30 seconds for 3 times.

33. Santolanasana variation 1: Same as Santolanasana with bent elbows, close to your body. Hold for 30 seconds for 3 sets.

34. Santolanasana variation 2: Sit in cat pose, straighten your knees move the shoulders forward push the buttock downwards until the body is straight and parallel to the floor. Slowly turn your full body to the right side and raise your left hand up shoulder level. Make sure your upper body weight is on your right hand and lower body weight on your left leg. Repeat the same with the other side. Hold for 20 seconds for 3 sets.

35. Suryanamaskar: 10 rounds, normally.

36. Suryanamaskar: 10 rounds with sit-ups. Do 5 sit-ups, then 1 Suryanamaskar. Repeat this for 10 rounds.

37. Ardha Chandrasana standing position: Feet together, hands by the side, put your right leg forward, bend your right knee at a 90-degree angle to the floor. Push your left leg behind till you feel the stretch on your left thigh, then inhale and raise your hands up in Namaskar Mudra with straightened elbows and arched back. Hold for 30 seconds with normal breathing. Repeat with the other leg for 3 sets each. This asana tones your thighs, butt, and your arms. It also stretches your abdominal and back muscles.

38. Naukasana: Inhale and raise both legs up, then raise

your upper body off the floor. Hold for 30 seconds while breathing normally. Repeat it for 5 sets. This asana tones your abdominal muscles and improves digestion and is also good for diabetes. Relax for 2 minutes after each set. Also, don't forget to do the counter pose (Kati Chakrasana) after each asana.

39. Side bending Chakrasana: While standing, put your feet together with your hands on the sides. Now raise your right hand up and stretch while bending your body towards the left side. Hold for 30 seconds, then come back to the original position. Repeat with the other side for 5 sets. This asana is beneficial to reduce fat from your love handles and arms, and is also good for asthmatic patients. It is also good for your side muscles.

40. Dhanurasana on the stomach: Lie on the floor on your stomach. Bend your knees, hold your ankles with your hands and inhale, while raising your upper body and your legs up, slowly. Hold for 15 to 20 seconds. Repeat it for 2 sets. This asana stretches your leg muscles, stomach, and back. If you have a severe back pain, please avoid this asana.

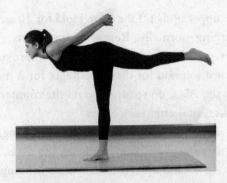

Ek Padasana (interlocking the hands at the back)

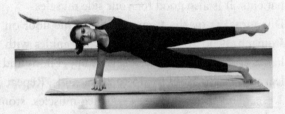

Ek Pada Hasta Santolanasana

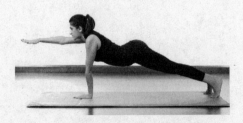

Santolanasana variation 1

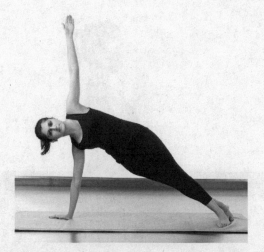

Santolanasana variation 2 (with one hand upwards)

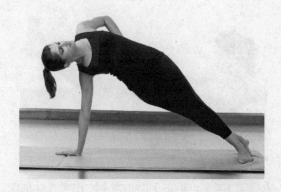

Santolanasana variation 3 (with one hand behind)

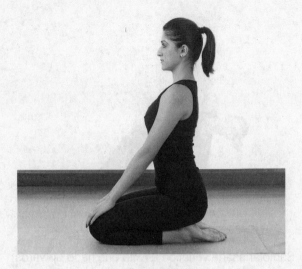

Vajrasana

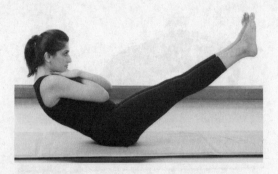

Naukasana variation 1 (hands across the chest)

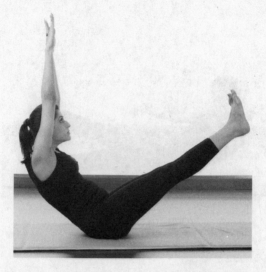

Naukasana variation 2 (with hands parallel to the ears)

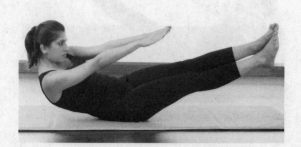

Poorna Triyak Naukasana

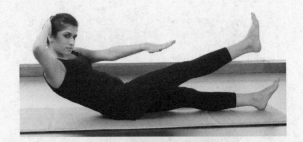

Ardha Triyak Naukasana

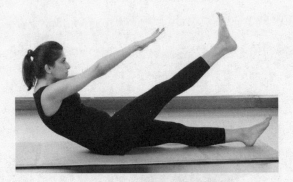

Ardha Naukasana

3

Fitness fundas

I first met Payal while we were shooting for *Golmaal 3*, in Ramoji Studios, in Hyderabad. She was on the sets with Kareena and I saw them working out together. They seemed to be really enjoying themselves while doing yoga, and it made me curious, so I thought I would give it a try. This is how I started doing yoga with Payal. Initially it was just for fun and I had my doubts whether I would be able to continue doing it. I have always been a very restless person and I had never imagined that yoga would work for me. Little did I know at the time that I would enjoy it so much; even get hooked.

I have always been health conscious and workout in a gym four days a week, so I have never had any weight issues. What I wanted was to work on my flexibility which is a very important component of fitness. And flexibility is something which only yoga can provide. After I started working with Payal, I feel I can stretch better. We exercise two days a week and I concentrate on improving my flexibility. I have also become calmer than before. Yoga was indeed an eye opener for me, and although I am still new to it, I feel it has made a difference already. I recommend it to all, even those who don't have any weight issues like me, and want to achieve new landmarks in fitness.

Tusshar Kapoor

Tusshar Kapoor's exercise routine

Age: 34   **Sessions: 1 hour, 2 days a week**

Target: Tusshar's workout is aimed, not at weight loss but at flexibility and feeling energetic.

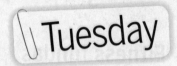

Tuesday

Start with warm up for 5 minutes
Suryanamaskars: 30 rounds

Standing positions:
1. Dandbetak: 30 sit ups, 3 sets
2. Trikonasana: hold for 20 seconds, repeat with the other side, 3 sets
3. Utkatasana: hold for 20 seconds, 3 sets
4. Side bending Chakrasana: hold for 20 seconds, each side, 3 sets
5. Tadasana: hold for 20 seconds, 3 sets
6. Vakrasana: hold for 20 seconds, 3 sets

Sitting positions:
7. Janu Shirshasana: hold for 20 seconds, each side, 3 sets
8. Paschimottanasana: hold for 20 seconds, 3 sets
9. Ustrasana: hold for 20 seconds, 3 sets
10. Marjariasana: hold for 10 seconds, 2 sets

Supine positions:
11. Setubandhasana: hold for 20 seconds, each side, 3 sets
12. Naukasana: hold for 20 seconds, 3 sets
13. Alternate elbow to knee movement: 20 times, each side, 3 sets
14. Ek Pada Ardha Halasana: hold for 20 seconds, 3 sets

Prone positions:
15. Sarpasana: hold for 10 seconds, 3 sets
16. Bhujangasana: hold for 10 seconds, 3 sets
17. Dhanurasana: hold for 10 seconds, 3 sets
18. Sahaj Pranayam: 10 rounds
19. Anulom Vilom: 10 rounds
20. Om chanting: 5 rounds
21. Breath consciousness while sitting: 5 minutes

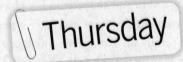

{ Yoga has made a huge difference to my level of fitness! }

Thursday

On Thursday, we mostly only stretch as Tusshar wants to work on his flexibility.

1 Spot jogging: 5 minutes
2 30 Suryanamaskars, slowly while concentrating on each posture

Standing positions:
3 Ardha Chandrasana: hold for 20 seconds, each leg, 2 sets
4 Parvatasana: hold for 20 seconds, each side, 2 sets
5 Trikonasana: hold for 20 seconds, each leg, 2 sets
6 Shishpadangustanasana: hold for 20 seconds, each leg, 2 sets
7 Vrikshasana: hold for 20 seconds, each leg, 2 sets

Sitting positions:
8 Janu Shirshasana: hold for 20 seconds, each side, 2 sets
9 Paschimottanasana: hold for 20 seconds, 2 sets
10 Pada Prasar Paschimottanasana sideways: hold for 20 seconds, each side, 2 sets
11 Pada Prasar Paschimottanasana forward: hold for 20 seconds, 2 sets
12 Ardha Matsyendrasana: hold for 20 seconds, each side, 2 sets

13 Ek Pada Ugrasana: hold for 20 seconds, 2 sets
14 Ugrasana: hold for 20 seconds, 2 sets

Supine positions:
15 Supta Vajrasana: hold for 10 seconds, 2 sets
16 Sarvangasana: hold for 20 seconds, 2 sets
17 Poorna Halasana: hold for 20 seconds, 2 sets
18 Saral Matsyasana: hold for 20 seconds, 2 sets

Prone positions:
19 Bhujangasana: hold for 10 seconds, 2 sets
20 Ardha Shalabhasana: hold for 10 seconds, each side, 2 sets
21 Poorna Shalabhasana: hold for 10 seconds, 2 sets
22 Sarpasana: hold for 10 seconds, 2 sets
23 Dhanurasana: hold for 10 seconds, 2 sets
24 Anulom Vilom Pranayam: 5 rounds
25 Kapalbhati: 25 strokes, 4 rounds
26 Om chanting: 5 rounds
27 Shavasana: 2 minutes

What is fitness?

Fitness, I feel, is one of the most misunderstood words. It does not mean having a slim and shapely body or having six packs. You can be at your ideal weight and have a perfect ten body and still not be totally fit. Fitness is a much broader term and includes important aspects of health like flexibility, stamina or endurance, strength, high energy levels, resistance to injuries that cause aches and pains, etc. It is a combination of qualities that enables the heart, lungs, muscles, etc., to perform at their full potential.

Monica Sharma, a 16-year-old student, is 5 feet 3 inches and weighs fifty-two kilos. She is young, slim, and attractive but cannot jog for even 2 kilometres. She starts panting and gets tired. On the other hand, her overweight mother Shalini Sharma at 44 years and sixty-one kilos can easily jog for 2 kilometres. So you see Shalini has more stamina than Monica even though she is older and heavier.

Fitness is important for everybody, but is especially important for those who have to do more physical work like sportsmen, actors, defence personnel, models, flight attendants, and fitness experts like me. It is especially important for sportsmen as their entire career depends on it. You must have heard of players not playing a match or a tournament as they were found to be unfit; Sania Mirza pulling out of a grand slam as she had some injury, or Sachin Tendulkar taking a break and working out to make his back stronger. Clearly, these people have no weight issues. So what are they striving for? Their goal is to be physically fit to be able to perform their best at the international level. So fitness is a step ahead of weight loss and a well-proportioned body. It is a lifelong challenge that we have to strive towards to enjoy life. Before we go any further, I would like you to take a basic fitness test I have designed to know your fitness level. This is something you can do at home on your own. Remember, you can lie but your body can't. ☺

How fit are you?

The first set of exercises test your cardio vascular endurance or the amount of oxygen being pumped into your heart and lungs.

1. Wear your running shoes and do spot jogging for 10 minutes. How long can you do it for?
   I. Less than 10 minutes
   II. Can do it for 10 minutes, but feel exhausted and breathless
   III. Complete 10 minutes and still feel energetic

   I use these exercises to test the functional capacity of the lungs. This test is recommended **for men and women in the age group of twenty to fifty years.**

2. How many times do you breathe in a minute?
   I. 15–25 times
   II. 10–15 times
   III. 5–8 times

3. Till how long can you hold your breath?
   I. 10–15 seconds
   II. 15–25 seconds
   III. 30–40 seconds

4. How long can you chant Om in one breath? Skip this exercise if you are pregnant or have heart problems or high blood pressure.

    I.   10–15 seconds

    II. 15–20 seconds

    III. 20–30 seconds

Through these exercises you can test your muscular endurance.

For men

1. How many push ups can you do at a stretch? Upper body
    I.   1–5
    II. 5–15
    III. 15–25

2. How many sit ups can you do in one go? Lower body
    I.   1–10
    II. 10–20
    III. 20–30

3. How many crunches can you do at a stretch?
    I.   1–10
    II. 10–25
    III. 25–50

For women

1. How many push ups on the knees can you do at a stretch? Upper body
    I.   1–5
    II. 5–15
    III. 15–25

2. How many sit ups can you do in one go? Lower body
    I.   1–10
    II. 10–20
    III. 20–30

3. How many crunches can you do at a stretch?
    I. 1–10
    II. 10–20
    III. 20–30

These three tests will help you determine the muscular strength of your body.

For men
1. Bend yourself like a chair (see p. 59). How long can you hold yourself like that?
    I. 10–20 seconds
    II. 20–30 seconds
    III. 30–40 seconds
2. Bring yourself in the push up pose with bent elbows. How long can you hold yourself like that?
    I. 1–10 seconds
    II. 10–15 seconds
    III. 15–30 seconds
3. Bend yourself like a boat with your middle touching the ground and your arms and legs in the air (see p. 66). How long can you hold yourself like that?
    I. 1–10 seconds
    II. 10–20 seconds
    III. 20–30 seconds

For women
1. Bend yourself like a chair (see p. 59). How long can you hold yourself like that?
    I. 5–10 seconds
    II. 10–20 seconds
    III. 20–30 seconds

2. Bring yourself in the push up pose with bent elbows. How long can you hold yourself like that?
   I.   1–5 seconds
   II. 5–10 seconds
   III. 10–20 seconds

3. Bend yourself like a boat with your middle touching the ground and your arms and legs in the air (Naukasana: see p. 66). How long can you hold yourself like that?
   I.   1–10 seconds
   II. 10–20 seconds
   III. 20–30 seconds

This exercise will tell you how flexible you are.

For men

1. Stand straight with your legs apart and then bend down (Pada Hastasana). How far do you reach without bending your knees?
   I.   shins
   II. ankles
   III. toes

For women

2. Stand straight with your legs apart and then bend down (Pada Hastasana). How far do you reach without bending your knees?
   I.   ankles
   II. toes
   III. toes and can touch your palms to the floor

Now it's crunch time. Want to know how well you've done? If you have:

11 IIIs: you are super fit
8–10 IIIs: you are fit
5–7 IIIs: you have average levels of fitness
Below 5 IIIs: your fitness levels are poor and you are unfit

Now that you know where you stand, you will be able to understand and appreciate the various parameters for fitness; like flexibility, stamina or endurance, strength, resistance to aches and pains, etc., better. By taking this test, you would've gotten to know your weak areas and what you should concentrate on. Fitness plays a crucial role in our daily life and overall health, and must not be ignored. Don't we all want to be fit to enjoy life? Play different kinds of sports, run on the beach, go trekking, hiking, walk for a stretch without panting and frantically searching for a chair. In this chapter, I will address these factors one by one, and suggest ways to improve upon them.

Flexibility

Have you ever admired the way Michael Jackson could twist and turn his body? Or closer home, how Hrithik sways almost effortlessly to those complicated dance sequences? This is because they are both extremely flexible. So what does flexibility really mean? Flexibility can be defined as the range of motions possible around a specific joint or muscle. Whether we walk, run, bend, or do any kind of movement, we need to use our joints and muscles, and the ease with which we can do it depends on how flexible we are. All body parts are not uniformly flexible. Like for example, some people might have a more flexible lower body while some others experience a greater flexibility in their upper body. Again, most people are more flexible on the right side of their body than the left. As a result, they find it easier to do any kind of exercise on their right side, but a little difficult on the left. Flexibility is especially important for athletes, sportspersons, actors, dancers, physical trainers, as well as all kind of performers. It is important for actors in Bollywood as they can do dance steps and actions scenes better if they are flexible.

For me flexibility is one of the most important factors fitness. Like I mentioned in my introduction, I was teased in school by my friends, who had nicknamed me 'rubberband', as I have been blessed with a highly flexible body. My body does not cramp easily; I can do exercises and yoga postures, even difficult ones, easily and my body recovers faster from injury.

How can I become more flexible?

Yoga offers several ways to improve flexibility. For starters, you can do regular stretching exercises, which keep the joints well lubricated and in turn more flexible. Other than that, there are some really simple ways to stretch any time during the day. Pull your hands backwards and on top of the head to unlock your muscles. You can do this while sitting as well as standing. It is good for your back, shoulders, and arms and will make you feel more energetic. You can also do counter poses after every thirty minutes or so. Like, if you have been sitting, bent forwards, working on your computer, you should pull your shoulder backwards to stretch your back. And these are such simple things that you can do them while commuting, standing in queues, cooking, watching TV, etc.

Although I have nothing against going to the gym, I have noticed that bodies of most gym goers are not flexible. This is mainly because they don't stretch after their workouts. Ideally, as I have already mentioned in chapter one, you should stretch before and after each workout, even if it is for 5 minutes. This not only prevents your muscles from cramping, but also improves blood circulation and flexibility.

I met Tusshar Kapoor a few months back while Bebo was shooting for *Golmaal 3*. He used to watch us exercise, and soon got tempted to try it out himself. Now Tusshar does not have any weight issues; he's slim and has a toned body as he has been going to the gym regularly for a long time. But he felt that he could improve on his dancing skills if he were more flexible. So I designed a special regime to help him achieve that. We now workout two days a week while he still goes to the gym four days. Tusshar is very disciplined with his workouts and I can already see improvements in his flexibility levels especially in the lower body. He has also become calmer than before.

Tips for feeling energetic in the morning

- Wash your face with ice cold water
- Listen to peppy or rhythmic music in the morning
- Do up your room in your favourite colours that cheer you
- Take your pet out for a walk
- Exercise in the morning

Saif's exercise routine

Age: 39 **Weight:** 75 kilos **Sessions:** 1 hour, 3 days a week
Target: To improve stamina, flexibility, and feel fresh.

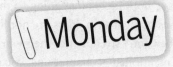

Monday

1 Warm up: 5–6 minutes
2 Suryanamaskar: 25 rounds for opening up of the body

Standing positions:
3 Side bending Chakrasana: hold for 30 seconds on the left and the right, each, 2 sets
4 Tadasana: hold for 20 seconds, 2 sets
5 Trikonasana: hold for 20 seconds on the left and the right each, 2 sets
6 Pada Hastasana: hold for 30 seconds, 1 set

Sitting positions:
7 Vajrasana: hold for 30 seconds, 2 sets
8 Uttan Mandukasana: hold for 10 seconds, 2 sets
9 Bhadrasana: hold for 30 seconds, 2 sets

Supine positions:
10 Supta Tadasana: hold for 10 seconds, 2 sets
11 Ek Padottanasana: hold for 30 seconds on the left and the right, each, 2 sets

12 Ardha Pavanmuktasana: hold for 30 seconds on the left and the right, each, 2 sets
13 Pavanmuktasana: hold for 30 seconds, 2 sets
14 Vipreetkarni: hold for 30 seconds, 2 sets

Prone positions:
15 Bhujangasana: hold for 30 seconds, 2 sets
16 Ardha Shalabhasana: hold for 10–30 seconds on the left and the right, each, 2 sets
17 Poorna Shalabhasana: hold for 10–30 seconds, 2 sets
18 Naukasana on the stomach: hold for 10 seconds, 2 sets
19 Dhanurasana: hold for 20 seconds, 2 sets
20 Makarasana: hold for 1 minute
21 Anulom Vilom Pranayam: 5 rounds
22 Jalandar Bandha: 3 rounds
23 Kapalbhati: 100 strokes, 4 rounds
24 Any auspicious chant: 3 rounds

> { Yoga is the best exercise I have done. The endorphines that dance around my brain after a class is something I haven't experienced before. }

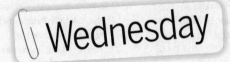

Wednesday

1. Warm up: 5–6 minutes
2. Suryanamaskar: 50 rounds
3. Trikonasana: hold for 30 seconds, each side, 2 sets
4. Ardha Baddha Padmottanasana: hold for 30 seconds, each side, 2 sets
5. Ardha Baddha Padmottanasana forward bending: hold for 30 seconds, each side, 2 sets
6. Ek Padasana: hold for 30 seconds, each side, 2 sets
7. Ek Padasana (interlocking fingers behind): hold for 30 seconds, each side, 2 sets
8. Ek Pada Ugrasana: hold for 30 seconds, each side, 2 sets
9. Ugrasana: hold for 30 seconds, 2 sets
10. Paschimottanasana: hold for 30 seconds, 2 sets
11. Ek Pada Uttan Paschimottanasana: hold for 20 seconds, each leg, 2 sets
12. Dwi Pada Uttan Paschimottanasana: hold for 20 seconds, 2 sets
13. Vakrasana: hold for 30 seconds, each side, 2 sets
14. Ardha Sarpasana: hold for 30 seconds, 2 sets
15. Sarpasana: hold for 30 seconds, 2 sets
16. Brahma Mudra: 2–4 rounds
17. Kapalbhati: 120 strokes, 3 rounds
18. Anulom Vilom: 12 rounds
19. Om chanting: 5 rounds
20. Shavasana: 2 minutes

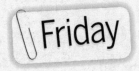

Friday

1 Warm up: 5–6 minutes
2 Suryanamaskar: 30 rounds
   (Suryanamaskar + 10 push ups)

Standing positions:
3 Trikonasana: hold for 25 seconds, 2 sets
4   Side bending Chakrasana: hold for 25
   seconds, 2 sets
5 Ardha Baddha Paschimottanasana:
   hold for 25 seconds, each leg, 1 set
6 Ardha Baddha Paschimottanasana
   (forward bending): hold for 25 seconds,
   each side, 1 set

Sitting positions:
7 Vakrasana sitting: hold for 25 seconds,
   2 sets
8 Ek Pada Uttan Paschimottanasana:

hold for 25 seconds, each side, 1 set
9 Dwi Pada Uttan Paschimottanasana:
   hold for 25 seconds, 1 set
10 Paschimottanasana: hold for
   25 seconds, 1 set
11 Parighasana: hold for 25 seconds, 1 set
12 Ek Pada Ugrasana: hold for 20 seconds,
   each side, 1 set
13 Uttan Mandukasana: hold for
   20 seconds, 2 sets
14 Ek Pada Vyaghrasana: hold for
   20 seconds, 1 set
15 Brahma Mudra: 2-4 rounds
16 Kapalbhati: 120 strokes, 3 rounds
17 Anulom Vilom: 12 rounds
18 Om chanting: 5 rounds
19 Shavasana: 2 minutes

Stamina or endurance

There are many forms of exercise to keep you fit; like weight resistance training, cardio vascular activity, kick boxing, mountain climbing, etc. The list, in fact, is unlimited. However, what all the above activities have in common is the requirement to push the body and the mind beyond the limits of endurance in order to break the mental and the physical barriers to achieve your goal. I have noticed that the discipline and the commitment to push the body and the mind, results in a similar approach to all spheres of life. Of all the various forms of exercise I have practised, I find yoga to be the most satisfying. It is a complete workout— mental and physical, internal, and external. The strength and determination required to complete a yoga class has to be tried to be 'believed'. If done in the right way as Payal trains, it is the definitive and the most complete of all workouts.

It is also important to exercise regularly so that you can maintain your fitness levels, and that does not only mean having a good body. Fitness is much more than that, and encompasses factors such as flexibility, stamina, and endurance. When I do yoga with Payal, it has a calming effect on my body, and I feel refreshed. I have been working out for the past two years with her, and I really enjoy it.

Saif Ali Khan

Whenever I think of fitness in terms of stamina and endurance, it reminds me of Saif, as he is one of the most energetic people I have ever come across. He has this unique ability of going on and on, and is able to juggle many things successfully. He is also extremely fit, and that I feel comes across in his personality and work. But then there are others who keep on complaining and don't feel like doing anything. 'I feel tired all the time!'; 'Can we do this tomorrow?'; 'What's the hurry?' are some of the common refrains that you will get from such people. Why is this so? One of the main reasons for such behaviour is that these people possess low stamina or the ability to continue working for a longer duration. And by work I mean both mental and physical work. They get tired easily and lack the energy to keep on going, in times of heavy workload. They lack the stamina which helps overcome fatigue or tiredness.

There are many reasons for having less stamina or not feeling up to something; some mental, others physical. It can be pure laziness that gradually becomes a habit, an excuse for when you're simply not interested, or even when you are afraid of taking responsibility. Strangely enough there are people who feel tired in the morning right after they wake up.

Rahul, my friend's husband, is a successful software analyst. He is around 40 years of age, and loves his job. Among our friends, we call him the computer wizard. Although Rahul loves his job, he feels very tired every morning. He would feel haggard and mentally tired. When I initially heard about this, I was a little confused. Usually, when you love your job, you never feel tired in the mornings. But then I found out the entire story. Rahul feels that he is not getting his due in his job. He has been working really hard for several years now but felt that his boss is taking him for granted, and not paying him enough. The peer pressure added to his worries especially when he saw less hardworking or talented colleagues doing much better professionally. And slowly but surely, it was eating him up. This was the root cause of Rahul feeling lethargic right in the morning. He was not satisfied with his job, and it reflected on his energy levels in the morning. However, there can also be physical causes for waking up with a frown in the morning. When you are not sleeping enough or have had a disturbed sleep, feel weak due to illness, have a bad hangover, feel stuck in a bad marriage, do not get enough sex, or even workout excessively, you can feel tired easily.

Energy drinks

There is a wide variety of energy drinks available in the market nowadays. Instant energizers are becoming increasingly popular among the youth. But instead of going for these artificial drinks which increase the heart beat in order to make you feel active, you should go for natural energy boosters like chilled watermelon juice, salt and sweet nimbu paani, sugarcane juice, lassi, etc., whenever you feel the urge for an energy drink.

Some people have the misconception that alcohol provides a spurt in energy while in reality it makes you feel drowsy as it decreases your pulse and numbs your nervous system. Too much of tea and coffee is also not good for health. In fact, having a lot of coffee over a period of time can cause anaemia.

Ways to enhance your stamina

Work for your own satisfaction

I had a colleague once who taught yoga with me in my studio Cosmic Fusion. She was just 22 years old, had a great body, and would always talk of becoming a model. Unfortunately, she had not yet got a good enough break in her modeling career. Since she was trained in it, she decided to teach yoga, but she could never get over her passion for modeling. She would constantly talk about her favourite models and designers and why she admired them so much. At times, she would look really lost and sad, and I almost felt sorry for her. She would also get tired very easily, and often bunk her classes. Her behaviour did irritate me a little as I felt she was not taking her work seriously. But it was not her casual attitude or laziness that was preventing her from giving her best. She simply did not enjoy her work.

It is very important for us to like and enjoy what we do. If you don't, then you'll end up feeling tired and miserable all the time. On the other hand, if you have the passion for your job, you'll always feel energetic and excited about it. Take for instance, Amitabh Bachchan. Even at his age, he works harder than his younger colleagues and puts them to shame by always being on time for his shoots. Surely, he can take it easy now, as he is a superstar. But passion for his work provides him the stamina to work longer and harder.

Manage your time well

Time management is very crucial in today's world. You need to prioritize things and do them in their order of importance.

All of us have to juggle so many things today—career, love, friends, hobbies, parents, etc.—that it's very easy to feel tired when you do not plan things well. Shahrukh Khan is known in the film industry for using his time really well. Despite being so busy and sought after, he finds time for everything and everybody. His schedule runs like clockwork and he is always in control of his time. And since he balances things so well, takes out time for work and play, he is always full of energy.

Nisha Malhotra, my client, is 25, slim and runs a restaurant business. She always compares herself with others and is fiercely competitive in everything she does. She is at her ideal body weight and does not need to lose any more kilos but she still wants to lose more weight. In fact, she is so obsessed with losing weight that she works out more than required and as a result feels weak and tired. What Nisha does not realize is that it is equally important for our mind and body to relax. Instead of over-exercising and worrying about others all the time, Nisha needs to find time to rest. Her low stamina is because she focuses only on work and denies herself any fun.

Don't save your energy: spend it to feel energetic

When Seema Kulkarni, a 36-year-old housewife came to me complaining about how tired she felt all the time, I was intrigued. Seema was just around three kilos overweight and had no medical history or temporary illness that would sap all her energy like she had described. I then asked her about her lifestyle. This got me the answer I was looking for. Seema had an army of servants—two full time, and five part time including her cook, driver, gardener, etc. She did supervise them all, but in terms of physical activity there was very little that she did. The nanny took care of the children and she would take a nap almost every day in the afternoon. Evenings were spent in front of the TV or in socializing. So it did not come as a surprise to me that Seema was feeling the way she did. Seema did not exercise at all neither did she exert her body in any way on a regular basis. This was the main reason for her feeling lethargic and tired all the time.

People do not realize how important it is to work to feel energetic. Most people who have high levels of stamina do some form of physical activity regularly even if it is walking in the evenings or mornings. Our body is like a machine and we need to use it to prevent it from rusting and getting old.

Do any form of physical exercise that you like be it gymming, aerobics, yoga, or simply jogging or running. You can also play any sport that you enjoy like, tennis, swimming, squash, kickboxing, cycling, etc. When we exercise, we sweat and the pores in our skin open up, releasing the toxins out of the body. It also improves the circulation of blood and oxygen supply to the various organs. After working out for two months, Seema is a changed person. She has lost the extra kilos and feels energetic and happy. She feels she can accomplish much more in a day than she used to before. I designed an hour-long workout for Seema, which she did five days a week, and still continues to do.

Strength

The last factor for fitness which we will talk about is strength.

What does strength mean? Strength is measured by the amount of force you can exert on a body, like when you push a trolley, lift a heavy shopping bag, or even open the cork of a bottle you display strength. All these activities require you to apply some force to execute them. While flexibility has a lot to do with the joints, strength is more closely related to the muscles in our body. The most common exercises for building strength are squats, lunges, push-ups, etc. In yoga you have specific exercises for building the strength in different muscles.

For building strength in the arms I recommend Parvatasana or the mountain pose. Legs can be made stronger by doing Utkatasana. It is very good for the toes, joints, and even the muscles of the feet. There are many different variations of Santolanasana that you can do for improving strength. For the abdominal area, I swear by Naukasana or the boat pose. When you are in Naukasana, your abdominal muscles are pressed, which helps in secretion of insulin and hence aids digestion. Doing Naukasana regularly will make your abdominal muscles strong, and then you can get that six pack much faster than others.

Aches and pains

All of us want to feel fit, agile, and healthy all the time. Aha! Wish this could be true in real life. Who likes to be confined to the bed and miss all the fun? We all want to make the most of life and do things that the others are doing—dancing, going out for movies, partying, etc. But life is not perfect nor are our bodies. It is normal to get hurt or fall ill occasionally. The only difference is that some of us are more prone to falling ill than others.

Aches and pain can be caused due to different reasons. Having a fall, or suffering sprains, and injuries is not in our control. It can be an accident or plain bad luck! These can result in concussions, fractures, etc. There are some other injuries that are caused due to misuse, overuse, or even under-use of body part. These can be prevented. You might have a weak back and still pick up some heavy luggage, or you might bend and pick up something from the floor with a jerk. These things should be avoided. Some other common ways in which we can inflict pain on ourselves is by having wrong postures, and using wrong chairs. If we sit tilted or stand bent for hours, it is no surprise that we end up having aches and pains in our body. Similarly, if you are fond of wearing stilettos or high-heeled shoes—you can damage your ankle.

In reality, aches and pains totally depend on the individual, the body type, body weight fitness, and strength. Besides these physical ones there can also be psychological origin to an ache. It has been proven that around 80 percent of all illnesses are psychosomatic in nature. This simply means that there is no material origin to these aches and pains, but they originate in the mind. There are some others who make pain a part of their lifestyle. They love to crib and complain about a joint pain or a back pain, and do nothing about it. They love their 'Ooh, aah, ouch' so much that sometimes even when they do not actually experience any discomfort, they would habitually feel it.

There are five basic things that you must do in case of any physical ache or pain:

1. Do not do any heavy exercises for five days.

In case you have a fresh injury, you should rest and let your body recover naturally. Do not do any form of exercise for at least five days, since your body needs time to heal first. If you workout despite an injury, there can be further wear and tear and it will worsen the injury.

2. Avoid sour foods.

Do not have any sour things till you heal. What happens is that the pain in your body is a result of the acids formed during the wear and tear of your muscle tissues. Now if you have sour things, which also contain acids, it will further aggravate your pain.

3. Drink milk or have calcium tablets.

To help your body recover fast and to provide it extra nourishment, drink a glass of milk with turmeric (haldiwala doodh) everyday till you get better. I would recommend you drink milk at room temperature as some people get acidity from hot milk while some others from cold milk. If you are not a milk drinker or are allergic to dairy products, you can have calcium tablets instead of milk.

4. Do hot and cold fomentation.

Fomentations are increasingly becoming popular all across the world. They are now being used in clinics, homes, spas, resorts, etc. Fomentations differ from compresses in that they are local applications of both hot and cold given alternately.

Compresses can also be hot or cold, but are not given alternately. Fomentations stimulate the circulation of blood in the body, aid in decongestion, soothe external tissue, and warm stiff joints. They can be used for acute inflammations, local pains and congestion, toothache, etc. For example, injuries while playing cricket in the legs, arms, etc., are mostly treated with cold fomentations instead of hot. In fact, injury is often treated by cold fomentations and jerks are treated through hot fomentations.

Cold fomentations should be applied to a fresh injury within 24 to 48 hours. It reduces blood circulation and restores any wear and tear. For a home based fomentation, place some cubes of ice in a handkerchief and apply on the affected area. You can also buy readymade compresses from the market and keep it in your fridge. Never do fomentations for more than 20 minutes at a time as it can damage your tissues. Tie with a crepe bandage and then elevate the foot.

Use hot fomentations for sprains and strains in your neck or back, or when you have a strain in your muscles like in your calf, groin, etc. It increases blood circulation in the area it is applied. You can do it at home using a hot water bag. Do it three to four times a day, and your pain will most likely be gone. Remember not to do it for more than 20 minutes at a time as it can damage your muscles.

5. Sleep well and rest.
This is one of the things that is often ignored after an injury or pain. People think that they can resume their life like normal after getting the basic treatment and a day's rest. But it might not be enough. The benefits of a good night's sleep and rest

are often underestimated. Sleep is very important to the healing process. It has an important role in physical healing, especially when you have sustained a muscle strain or any other kinds of injury.

Now let's talk about some common types of aches and pains.

Injury while playing sports

When you play any form of sport, be it cricket, hockey, football, or tennis, you have to be more fit than normal. In fact, physical fitness is extremely crucial in a sportsperson's career. Your body undergoes more wear and tear and you are more prone to injuries. Sportspersons are generally most prone to ankle and hamstring injuries. Football and hockey players have to watch out for their back, whereas there is a greater chance of injuries in the quadriceps and calf muscles while playing tennis and basketball. Interestingly, swimming is probably the only sport in which you don't normally suffer any injuries.

What to do? Well, you cannot really be completely injury free. It is a part of our life and we have to accept it whether we like it or not. However, you can do regular stretching exercises and yoga asanas to increase your flexibility and enhance the resistance to injuries. Consult your physiotherapist and do not skip your stretching and workout sessions. You should also not underestimate the importance of adequate rest for the body. And yes, cut down on your drinking while playing or when your tournament is on.

Pain in the head

Headaches are the most common kind of aches. Most of us have accepted it as a part of our existence, and hence we just pop a pill and forget about it. But do you know why we get headaches? There are three main reasons for headaches—cold, mental tension, and constipation. And there is a simple way I use to find out the cause of your headache. If you have a headache due to cold, you will feel the pain mostly on your forehead; tension causes pain in the back of the head while if the headache is due to constipation, you will feel the pain on the right side of your head. Some other causes of pain in the head are low blood pressure, irregular food habits, lack of sleep, weak eyesight, PMS in women, strong odours, sinusitis, injury, other medical conditions, etc. I remember how I got a severe headache when I had gone to Tirumala in Andhra Pradesh, and was standing in long queue for hours for the darshan. There were thousands of eager devotees like me all around and we were waiting for our turn to get one glimpse of the deity, Balaji.

You might have noticed that you get headaches in buses, crowded or smoke-filled places, temples, centrally air conditioned places like malls, aircrafts, etc. These congested places reduce the oxygen supply to the brain through the blood flow, and cause headaches.

Pain in the neck

The neck is one of the most delicate and critical parts of your body. It connects our head with the rest of the body and it is here that many important glands like thyroid, parathyroid, etc., are located. Under ideal conditions, the neck should be aligned with the back.

There are both internal and external factors for pain or discomfort in the neck. Internal factors can be cold, cough, tonsillitis, cervical spondylosis, etc. External causes constitute lifting weights, excessive exercise, jerks, using the wrong kind of mattresses or pillows, and so on. Any of these can give your neck a tough time. I still remember the time in college when my cousins had planned a sleepover at my place and we ended up watching *Scream 2* at night. To create the right atmosphere we had switched off all lights and kept the windows open. There was complete silence in the room as we were all concentrating hard on what was going to happen next. Just then, the door opened and my mom entered the room. My cousin, Neha, who was sitting next to the door got up with a start and the sudden jerk on her neck resulted in a severe sprain! We haven't watched scary movies together since.

I have often noticed that people working in the service industry like hotels, airlines, etc., complain of pain in the neck and the spine. They have to stand for long hours, and keep running around to make sure things are in order. As a result, their neck and back get affected easily.

Pain in the back

Our back or spine is like the pillar on which the entire body rests. But the strongest part can also be the weak spot if not taken care of well. Backaches can be due to the bones as well as the muscles. Most commonly, the pain in the back is due to the strain in the spinal rectus muscles attached to the spine and not the spine itself. Slip disc, cervical problems, spondylosis, lumbar spondylosis, overgrowth of bones, etc., are causes of backache due to the spine.

Here again, there can be internal as well as external causes for it. Internal causes can be pain in the pelvic region or pelvis, gastroenteritis, chest pain, constipation, kidney problems, etc. Sprains are one of the main external causes for backaches.

Gulshan Kaur is a 37-year-old housewife. She has always been very fitness conscious, and would love to hit the gym regularly. Unfortunately, once while she was picking up weights in the gym, her back snapped, and she was advised by the doctor not to pick up any weights for forty-five days. After taking the recommended break, when Gullu resumed gymming, she realized that even with a little twitch her back would get dealigned, which would hurt her a lot. And it was not only while exercising, she had to be careful at home too. Her back would get de-aligned even while doing any kind of regular household work. Confused and worried, Gullu came to me and started doing yoga, especially exercises to strengthen her back. Now the frequency of her back pain has substantially reduced and it occurs only around once in six months. Gullu loves what yoga has done to her body, and believes with regular practice, her back problem will go away forever.

Other common causes for backache include using the wrong mattress to sleep on. Your mattress should neither be too soft nor too hard. At your workplace, make sure you use a comfortable chair with a backrest. Most of us with a desk job spend hours at a stretch sitting on the chair; and it is extremely important that you use the right kind of chair to avoid recurring back pain. Bad postures are also responsible for backaches. Some people have the habit of driving with the chair pushed tilted back, which also induces backache.

Drooping shoulders, sitting in a sloppy manner or with a

bent back, watching TV lying on the bed or the sofa, carrying a heavy load on your back like a school bag, laptop, shopping bags or side slinging bulky bags which apply pressure only on one side of the shoulder, wearing high heels, etc. can also cause back aches if continued on a regular basis. Don't carry

Tips for working for long hours on the computer

- Sit erect
- Check your posture after every 15 minutes
- Use the right kind of chair with good back support
- Rotate your neck every 2 hours
- Don't sit or stand for long hours at a stretch
- Do counter poses; arch your back 2 to 3 times in a day
- Twist your back left and right
- Your screen should be at your eye level
- Don't bend forward too much while working

your laptop on one side while walking. Keep shifting it from one shoulder to the other. If you mostly wear the same formal shoes to work, chances are that after three to four months, one side will get worn out more than the other. So you should try and replace such shoes, as an uneven walk causes back pain. Also, you should try and avoid walking on irregular surfaces or slopes, especially in high heels, as this could lead to spraining your back, if not your ankle.

A sudden gain of weight, obesity, or beer bellies can also cause backaches as you are forcing the back to carry more

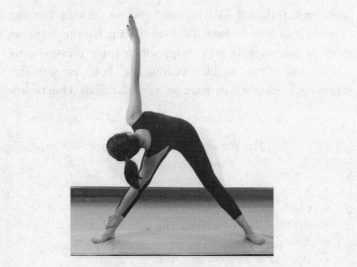

Trikonasana

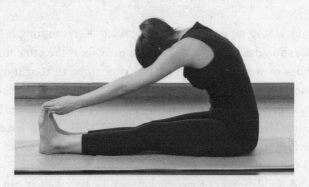

Paschimottanasana

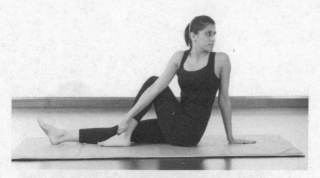

Vakrasana

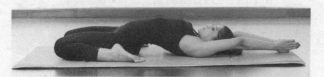

Supta Tadasana

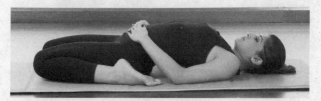

Supta Vajrasana

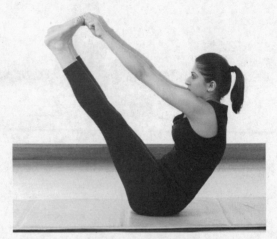

Dwi Pada Uttan Paschimottanasana

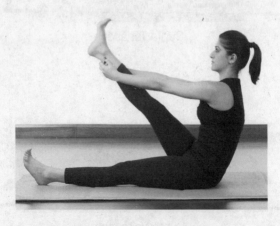

Ek Pada Uttan Paschimottanasana

weight than it should.

Yoga routine for working people

This is a workout that I especially recommend for working people. Whether you work at the desk or your job involves standing for hours, the areas that get most affected are your back, neck, and shoulders. This exercise routine is beneficial for people with chronic backache and also helps relieve pain in the neck and the shoulders. Try it for three months and you will experience the difference.

Precaution: In case you have acute backache, don't do Kapalbhati but you can do the rest of the exercises.
Duration: 35 to 40 minutes
Ideal time: In the morning after going to the loo or if you want to do it in the evenings, then 4 hours after lunch or 1 hour before dinner; do it three times a week.

1. Lying in supine position
   - Supta Tadasana: hold for 20 seconds
   - Ek Pada Uttanasana: hold for 30 seconds on the right and the left leg each, 1 set
   - Crocodile series: 3 minutes
   - Ardha Pavanmuktasana: hold for 30 seconds on the right and the left leg each, 1 set
   - Pavanmuktasana: hold for 30 seconds, 1 set
2. Lying in prone position
   - Makarasana: 1 minute
   - Bhujangasana: hold for 30 seconds, 1 set

- Makarasana: hold for 30 seconds
- Ardha Shalabhasana: hold for 20 seconds on the right and the left side each, 1 set
- Niralambasana: 1 minute, 1 set
- Makarasana: hold for 30 seconds, 1 set
- Naukasana on the stomach: hold for 10 seconds
- Makarsana: hold for 30 seconds, 1 set

3. In sitting position
   - Vakrasana: hold for 30 seconds on the right and the left side each, 1 set
   - Brahma Mudra: 3 rounds
4. Kapalbhati: 50 strokes, 3 rounds
5. Anulom Vilom Pranayam: 5 rounds
6. Shavasana: breathe 50 times slowly with breath consciousness

Pregnant? Watch your back

- Sleep on your side with a pillow under your stomach
- When you wake up, don't get up straight, turn on your side, and then get up.
- Use a good mattress to sleep on.
- Sit in the kitchen and work; don't tire yourself by standing for long hours.
- You need to do special prenatal exercises; don't follow your regular routine.
- Don't lift anything heavy.
- Take extra calcium and protein in your diet.

Pain in the limbs

What is the role of the limbs in our body? Arms help to balance the body, and are used in most of our daily chores like writing, typing, lifting something, talking on the phone, playing games, driving, cooking, etc. Arms include joints like the shoulders, elbows, wrists as well as muscles such as biceps, triceps, forearm flexors, etc.

Legs are the most important and the most ignored part of our body. Legs includes the entire lower body like the gluteus muscles, thigh joints, quadriceps, hamstring, knee joints, calf muscles, ankle joints, etc. Even though they are always active and take on the weight of the entire body, we often do not pay much attention to them.

Aches and pains in the limbs can be due to wear and tear or any kind of problem with the joints. Overuse of the joint makes it more susceptible to injuries. The three most common kinds of injuries to the arms are:

Frozen shoulders

Frozen or stiff shoulders can cause persistent pain and are often the result of wrong exercise or lifting excessive weight. Frozen shoulders result in immobility or stiffness, and you might feel as if your arms are locked, sometimes even preventing you from lifting them.

Tennis elbow

Tennis elbow, as the name suggests, is mainly found in tennis players. It is caused due to weak muscles or injury while playing cricket, squash, or tennis. Even our master blaster

Sachin has had complaints of a tennis elbow.

Wrist sprain

Wrist joints are one of the most active joints as we use them extensively, for our daily work. They are also very sensitive especially in women, and can be sprained or dislocated easily. People with arthritis experience pain in their wrists as they become stiff for lack of adequate lubrication. You should be careful while lifting heavy baggage so that your wrist does not snap.

The three most common types of injuries to the legs are:

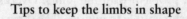

Tips to keep the limbs in shape

- Keep the joints busy and active; activities such as swimming, running, biking cycling, climbing stairs, and dancing are good for your limbs.
- Exercise regularly but don't overdo it.
- Rotate the shoulders, elbows, wrists, knees, ankles, etc., to open up the joints.
- Flex and extend the elbows regularly.
- Apply hot or cold fomentations for injuries.
- Stretching your biceps, triceps, and deltoid muscles make them more flexible.
- Strengthen your biceps, triceps, and forearms through yoga postures.
- Include protein and calcium in your diet. So don't shy away from eating soyabean, eggs, meat, chicken, fish; and dairy products like milk, paneer, cheese, etc.

Hamstring hazards

Pain in the hamstring is most common in sportspersons as well as some other people. Cricketers often strain their hamstrings while fielding and chasing the ball. You must have noticed the physiotherapist running on to the field and applying cold fomentation. Hamstring can hurt when we overuse them and even when they are less utilized than they should be.

Knee problems

The knee is a condylar joint and reacts when we ignore or misuse it. Pain in the knee is mostly due to applying excess pressure on it due to obesity, or running on the treadmill for more than 30 minutes. The delicate knee cartilage gets worn out due to jumping excessively on your heels or even while driving a bike as it causes repeated jerks in the area.

Ankle twists

Ankle woes are very common nowadays. Injuries to the ankles can be caused due to wearing high heels, standing for long hours at a stretch. This can be cured with hot and cold fomentation within 48 hours of the injury, and even resting it from time to time.

Women woes

Manya Talwar is a 17-year-old college going girl who has had complaints of very heavy and painful periods since the time she started having them. Manya had accepted this as a part of her life but now that she is thinking of training as a commercial pilot, she did not want it to come in the way of her performance. She did not want to pop pills throughout her life, as she was worried that it might cause complications later on.

She came to me worried and desperately looking for a natural solution. I worked with Manya for three months, and now she does the workout I prescribed, on her own. Her periods have become regular and less painful, and she's dreaming of conquering the skies without fear or worry.

Well, periods are an integral part of our growing up, and all of us have to live with them, it even though we would at times wish they would disappear. While some of us have regular, almost painless periods, the rest of us are not so lucky and experience painful cramps, dizziness, bloating, etc.

We women do have some specific problems, and here is one workout that I have designed especially for all of us. This workout is useful in dealing with irregular periods, excessive bleeding, very painful cramps, etc.

Workout for specific female problems like heavy blood flow during periods, irregular or painful periods, polycystic ovaries (PCOD), and excess weight on the abdomen.
Duration: 1 hour ideally, but do only as much as you can without exerting your body.

Ideal time: The best time to do this workout is in the morning after going to the loo. However, if you want to do it in the evenings, then start 4 hours after lunch or one hour before dinner. Do it three times a week, and you will feel the difference in a couple of months.

Start with a warm up of 5 minutes

Kapalbhati: 50 strokes, 4 rounds

1. Standing positions
   - Side bending Chakrasana: hold for 30 seconds on the right and the left, 2 sets
   - Konasana: hold for 30 seconds, 2 sets
   - Kati Chakrasana: hold for 30 seconds, 2 sets
   - Pada Hastasana: hold for 30 seconds, 2 sets
   - Tadasana: hold for 20 seconds, 2 sets
2. Sitting positions
   - Vajrasana: hold for 30 seconds, 1 set
   - Parvatasana in Padmasana: hold for 30 seconds, 2 sets
   - Vakrasana: hold for 30 seconds on the right and the left, 2 sets
   - Bhadrasana: hold for 30 seconds, 2 sets
   - Bhadrasana with forward bending: hold for 30 seconds, 2 sets
   - Ugrasana: hold for 30 seconds, 2 sets
3. Supine positions
   - Shavasana: 2 minutes
   - Supta Tadasana: hold for 10 seconds
   - Ek Pada Uttanasana: hold for 30 seconds on the right; 30 seconds on the left, 2 sets
   - Crocodile variation: series 1, 2, 3, 4
   - Ardha Halasana: hold for 30 seconds, 2 sets
   - Ardha Pavanmuktasana: hold for 30 seconds on the right; 30 seconds on the left, 2 sets
   - Pavanmuktasana: hold for 30 seconds, 2 sets
   - Supta Bhadrasana with Mula Bandha: 5 rounds
4. Prone positions
   - Bhujangasana: hold for 30 seconds, 2 sets

- Ardha Shalabhasana: hold on the right and left sides for 30 seconds each, 2 sets
- Poorna Shalabhasana: hold for 30 seconds, 2 sets
- Naukasana: hold for 20 seconds, 2 sets
- Dhanurasana: hold 20 seconds, 2 sets.

5. Brahma Mudra: 1 round
   - Bhastrika: 4 rounds
   - Anulom Vilom Pranayam: 5 rounds
   - Bhramari: 5 rounds
   - Om chanting: 5 rounds

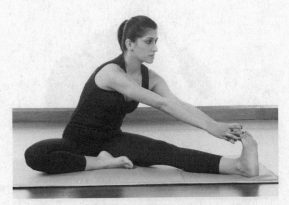

Ek Pada Ugrasana

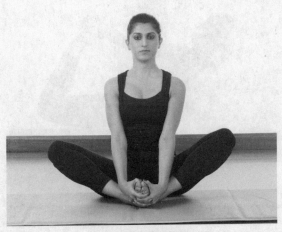

Bhadrasana

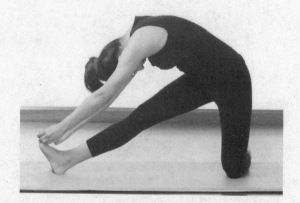

Parighasana

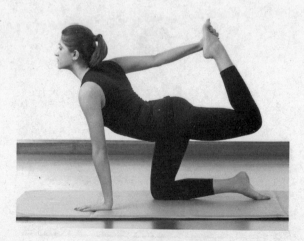

Ek Pada Vyaghrasana

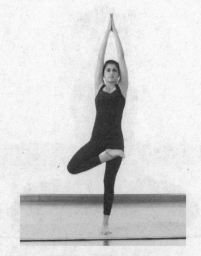

Ardha Baddha Padmmothanasana

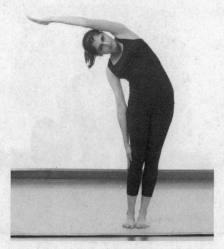

Side bending Chakrasana

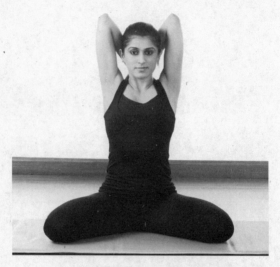

Uttan Mandukasana

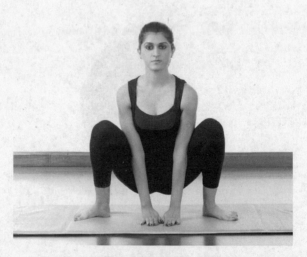

Uttanasana

4

How to put it together

I have said it right at the beginning of the book, and I will repeat myself here again. *From XL to XS* is a practical guide to fitness, and it is really important for me that my readers should be able to read the book, and apply the things that I talk about in their daily lives. That is the reason I have given complete and detailed workouts, including things like what you might need while exercising, basic precautions, the time duration, benefits, etc., so that you know how to go about it. I want people to read the book and actually use it to look good rather than keep it back on their shelves. The first three chapters in the book deal with three separate issues—weight loss, changing the shape of your body and becoming a perfect ten, and improving your fitness level. As I can imagine, there will be three kinds of people who will use this book:

1. People who have never exercised, and want to lose weight.

2. People who have been working out and have no weight issues but rather want to use the book to change the shape of their body, which only yoga can help them achieve. They might also want to work on some particular aspect of fitness; be it flexibility, stamina, or strength.

3. People who are already doing yoga, cardio vascular exercises, pilates, playing any kind of sport or going to

the gym, and might not need to change the shape of their body but might be interested in fitness or any specific area in fitness.

How can these different sets of people use the workouts in this book?

Beginners who want to lose weight can refer to chapter one and achieve their ideal body weight by following the workout as per the category they fall into. So if you are twelve kilos overweight, you can follow case study 2, and get slim. A lot of people get lax after they have lost the number of kilos that they wanted to and stop exercising. However, this is when you need to be extra cautious. Let me ask you something. Do you stop eating after losing weight? Of course not! So if you are consuming calories, you need to exercise as well to burn them out. And if you don't, then you will be back to where you started. If you want to enjoy life to the fullest, make exercise a part of your regular routine, just as breathing, sleeping or eating is. So my advice to you would be to carry on with the workout for beginners given at the end of the book to maintain your weight. By following this workout, you will be able to maintain your weight and improve your overall fitness at the same time. In case you want to change the shape of your body, you can then add the regimes in Chapter 2 as per your body shape to your regular workout. So if you are apple shaped, do your regular workout six days a week and then, on three days, add the workout for the apple shape to your regular workout. For example, I feel Tuesdays, Thursdays, and Saturdays are lighter days for me in terms of my workload. So if I want to change the shape of my body, I would follow the shapes' regime after my regular workout on these days.

For people who have already been doing some form of exercise like yoga, pilates, gymming, etc., and do not really need to lose weight, it is advisable that they continue with what they are doing and add the shapes regime to it. So for all shapes, except the ball-shaped physique, you can add your shapes regime to your regular workout and do it three times a week. For the ball shape, you need to follow the workout every day, and do it after whatever form of exercise you are doing. In case, you are interested in only one aspect of fitness, you can add those specific exercises to your existing routine and do it three times a week.

The workouts routines of all the stars in the book cater to all the three aspects of fitness mentioned in the first three chapters—weight loss or maintaining their weight, changing the shape of your body and becoming a perfect ten, and working on various fitness parameters like stamina, strength, and flexibility. They might focus one or two particular aspects but they cover all. So if you are the same shape as the star, then you can follow their regime and not do anything else. If you are doing nothing else, then just follow the regimes, six days a week for all aspects. But do this only after you have achieved your ideal body weight.

Part Two

In the Mind

5

How to look ten years younger

How do I manage to look young? Aah…it's a secret! Just kidding ☺!

For me the most important thing is doing things in moderation. I believe you can do whatever you like, eat or drink whatever you want, and still look much younger than your age if you do all of these within a certain limit. Another thing, which I feel is really important is using as little make-up as possible in daily life. You must be really disciplined about your beauty regime as soon as you hit 25. Cleanse your skin regularly, use a good moisturizer diligently, and get a good night's sleep. Otherwise, your skin will wrinkle sooner, making you look old and haggard. And of course, physical activity is as important. I have been doing yoga since the past seven years, and this is the favourite time of my day, which I do not want to miss at any cost. I feel young and fresh after my workouts. The last, but most important thing, I would say is being happy, and cultivating hobbies. I took up painting recently, and I really enjoy this time alone with myself. Try my tips and you too might look younger than your age.

Sridevi

In the first part of the book we talked about how to get a beautiful body—how to lose weight, change the shape of our body, and stay fit. We have already talked at length about all physical aspects of our body. Now in the second part, we will discuss some invisible yet vital factors like ageing, beauty, sleep, and stress which play an almost silent yet significant role in determining how we look. Let's start with talking about something that bothers all of us at one stage or the other of our lives—growing old.

Are you in your mid-twenties? If yes, then wake up! Age is catching up with you, and it is high time that you do something about it. In today's times, if you have crossed 25, you need to start taking ageing seriously. You can see visible signs of ageing already creeping up if you look closely at yourself. So the sooner you start taking care of your youth, the better it is.

What happens when you are 25 plus? Most of the women these days get married after they cross 25 (and not in their early twenties like a few decades back), and enter a totally new phase in their lives. With marriage, comes additional responsibilities. You have to take care of your home, husband, children, family, etc., besides your work and your own sets of friends. The truth is that you're no longer a proverbial 'free bird' as you would say. If as a single woman you never had to bother about relatives, friends and family, now you have two sets of families and two sets of friends to manage. As they say, in India, a marriage is not only between a couple, but also between their families. I like to think it involves friends too.

What does this mean? In short, you have to socialize more than before, and have more things and people to deal with—so many more birthdays, anniversaries, weddings, parties, etc.

You also have different kinds of roles to play. You may be wife one second, mother the other, and daughter-in-law the next moment. Sounds tough, doesn't it? Most women get lost in this milieu and tend to ignore their own needs—the needs of their own mind and body. Indian women always tend to give preference to their husbands, children, and families. And it's not only your home that you have to deal with. If you work, then your list is longer. You have to deal with work pressure, deadlines, competition, office politics, etc.

I'm not saying that this is wrong or you should not do it. In fact, the first and foremost thing is to accept it as an unchangeable reality of your life. Second, find a way to handle it. Cribbing about it all the time will make no difference except taking a toll on your body and accelerating your ageing process.

I got married just a year and a half ago and I have myself experienced the sweeping changes that come in a woman's life after she gets married. However, even if you are single, there are greater work responsibilities that you have to handle besides your love life. In reality, it is not as difficult if you have the right approach. I have found a way to deal with it successfully, and I want to share this secret with you. All of us have to go through this phase and you just have to get mentally and physically prepared to handle it well. What I follow myself, is what I recommend to you: twenty-three hours for others; one hour for yourself. Isn't that workable? Surely, you can take out around one hour for yourself in a day! And believe me, you just need an hour to take care of your body. It has worked for me and it will work for you too! However, if you do not wake up in time you might be

one of those who age early, and look as old as they are if
not older.

What is ageing?

Ageing is a natural process—something that all of us have to
go through. But it is also true that none of us want to look
old and haggard. Youth is priceless and we want to hold on
to it for as long as possible. Consequently, we always look for
ways to delay ageing as much as possible. And why not? Who
doesn't want to look younger?

But let us first understand what ageing really means and
what it does to our body. As we grow older, our internal and
external organs become weak and less efficient. The metabolic
rate of the body slows down, supplying less oxygen to the body
parts. As a result, our organs feel exhausted, overworked, and
not as well maintained as they used to be. Our taut skin begins
to sag, fine lines start appearing on our face, our stamina
reduces, and we feel tired sooner than we would in our teens
or twenties. This is the truth of our existence, but in today's
times we do many things consciously or unconsciously which
accelerate the ageing process. What should have happened at
forty, now happens at 30 or even 25.

The other day I met a lady who is just 23 years old but
looks like a 42 year old woman. But at the same time, there
are others who, like Sridevi, look much younger than their
age. She not only has a lovely face, supple skin, and a slim and
fit body, but also has that inner glow, which makes her look
calm and beautiful. You too can look ten years younger than
your real age. If you lead the right lifestyle, and do the right
things at the right time, it is possible to look much younger

than you actually are. However, if you just go with the flow and ignore your own body, it will start ageing very soon.

What are the signs of ageing?

Our physical appearance or our outer body is a reflection of what's happening inside. If we are healthy from inside, it shows, and vice versa. Your face mirrors your age, and it is here that the first signs of ageing develop.

It's simple: you can make out how old a person is by his or her face. You start developing fine lines around your eyes, get dark circles, and laughter lines around your mouth. Next is your neck, which starts wrinkling especially if you have a dry skin. The other parts of your body which easily reveal your age are the skin of your hands and your feet. The skin of your hand may become loose, showing the veins and you may develop crow's feet, a sign of advanced age.

The second most significant change that ageing brings about is with respect to the postures. There is a marked difference in our postures as we age. You might have noticed that an older person cannot stand erect, has drooping shoulders, needs a chair and cannot sit on the floor or sit cross legged or for long hours, etc. Here I am reminded of Sunita Jain, who is a 56-year-old advertising professional. She has always led a very active life, balancing her work and family well. But since the past two years or so, since she retired from her job, she finds it very difficult to sit cross legged on the floor as her knees cannot bend. Unlike before, when she now goes for pujas or jagarans she has to sit on a chair with the other older ladies.

Some other signs of ageing are, sudden hair fall and

Menopause and andropause

What is menopause? When the ovaries in women stop producing eggs it leads to a gradual end of the menstrual cycle. This is referred to as menopause and happens usually around the age of 45 to 50 years. It indicates the advent of old age, when you can no longer have babies, and also causes hormonal changes in the body. The most common symptoms of menopause are sudden mood swings, irritability, irregular bowels, hot flushes, night sweat, vaginal dryness, fatigue, weight gain, memory loss, bloated stomach, heavy or low flow, loss of libido, etc. These days some women have it much earlier due to diet and lifestyle changes.

What is andropause? Even men have andropause when the testosterone levels in their bodies go down. It usually starts around the age of 45 but accelerates after 50 years. It is not only with women. Men, too, undergo changes in their bodies as they age. The most common symptoms of andropause are erectile dysfunction, listlessness, lack of libido, irritability, mood swings, depression, sleep disorder, rapid balding, etc.

Menopause or andropause is something that you cannot avoid. Everybody has to go through it sooner or later so it is better to know what it is and learn how to cope with it. The people around the menopausal or andropausal men or women especially their partners, family, children, etc., need to be very understanding as the hormonal changes can lead to mood swings and sudden unexpected reactions. But remember that this is just a temporary phase that will tide over soon. There is nothing medically wrong with them, and what they need is just your love and support.

greying, memory loss, headaches, irritable bowels, excessive appetite, stiff or immobile joints, early menopause, etc. Since the bone density decreases with age, you are more prone to diseases such as osteoporosis, arthritis, etc. The overall frame of your body looks crouched or stooped. Similarly, the muscles become weak and shrunken, and make you look crouched and stunted.

The last but most devastating sign of ageing may be the early advent of chronic diseases such as asthma, heart ailments like hypertension or high blood pressure, diabetes, and insomnia followed by lung and kidney diseases. All these are ways for your body to tell you that you are growing old. Who wants to look old and worn out and that too while still young? If this happens sooner than it should, like in your twenties or thirties, you cannot enjoy life to its fullest. On the other hand, if you can delay ageing, you can take pleasure in the small as well as big things that life offers, for much longer.

My six principles to look ten years younger

Many people I meet are surprised when I tell them that I am 35 years old. They often tell me, 'Payal, you look so young. How do you do it?' Interestingly, now instead of hiding my age, I like sharing my age with people, and seeing their reactions. I am sure Sridevi too gets a lot of that. Well, it's not difficult. Doesn't she look gorgeous and at her age? You can also look ten years younger than you are.

Over the years, working with my clients, I have developed my own principles for looking young and fresh. And I want to share it with all of you through this book. My six principles for looking younger are simple, inexpensive, and something that you can do on your own. However, all of these principles are equally important, and to experience the results, you must follow all diligently. There are no half measures and don't think that you can pick out what you like and leave the rest. If you follow a few of the principles, and not the rest you may not get the desired results. Also, the sooner you start the better it is. I feel as soon as you cross 25, you should be vigilant about ageing and follow these principles to remain young for much longer. And this is a very small price to pay to look like your daughter's sister or your friend's daughter!

Principle 1: Drink 4 litres of water everyday

My first rule is about drinking the right amount of water. You must drink at least 4 litres of water every day without fail. You can drink more than this if you like, but certainly not less. Suresh Nair, a colonel in the army, has been drinking at least 5 litres of water every day since his childhood. As a result, even at forty-eight, he has clear skin and good digestion, which makes him look much younger than his colleagues. This was inculcated in him by his mother and he feels really lucky to have developed this habit.

How is water important for preventing ageing? What does water do? About 70 percent of our body is made up of water. Water is the natural lubricant of your body, and works with your metabolism. It keeps the skin soft and hydrated, and the body light by removing the toxins from our system. With the help of the kidney, water filters the harmful chemicals in the blood out of the body, and cleanses it. But if you do not drink sufficient amounts of water, your blood thickens, and you are more prone to heart diseases.

Most people do not know that there are three ways of providing life-giving oxygen to the body—through the air in the atmosphere, pores in the body, and water that we drink. So remember whenever you are drinking water, you are also helping your body breathe.

What happens when you do not water your body as required? First, you may suffer from regular constipation or irregular bowel movements, and feel heavy and bloated all the time. Second, since the toxins remain in your body, they will slowly but surely start reflecting on your skin. Your skin might develop acne, boils, patches, spots, etc. Third, your eyes might dry up, and you would have to strain your eyes to watch TV, etc. Fourth and most important, your blood might thicken, making your metabolism rate go down. You may also complain of low blood pressure, as a result of your blood thickening, and the lack of sufficient fluids in your body.

What is the solution? Simple—drink 4 litres of water every day. It will prevent toxins from accumulating in your body, and throw them out of your system regularly. The results can be seen in your skin, hair, eyes, nails, digestion, etc. Refer to the water chart in chapter one to drink 4 litres of water each day.

Principle 2: Must have 1 tablespoon flax seeds each day

The second rule that I have is about your diet. It is not only important to drink the right amount of water, but also to eat the right kind of food to look younger. Most of us know that we should eat regularly and in small quantities. We should lead a routine life, avoid smoking, drinking and drugs. Alcohol and drugs slow down your metabolic rate, and accelerate ageing. Nitin Mishra, a 23-year-old software professional, is a chain smoker, smoking almost thirty cigarettes in a day. He has been smoking for the past five years and now his teeth are a dark yellow, his eyes puffy and groggy, his face bloated, with very dull looking skin. Although he is just 23, he looks like he is in his mid-thirties. Smoking and drugs are especially bad for the skin, and makes it look dry and papery. Tobacco also stains your teeth and, with prolonged use, turns them into that unattractive yellow, which all of us are familiar with.

We should also avoid white foods like maida, sugar, junk food, fried foods, coloured foods, etc., that are difficult to digest, and harmful for the body. What is it, then, that you should eat to look younger? You must have 1 tablespoon of

Things to not eat to prevent ageing

- Fried food such as pakoras, samosas, vada pao, fries, puris, etc., should be avoided. But if you really crave it, then have it once a week, but make sure that the oil does not have trans-fat.
- White food like maida, breads, pastry, patties, pasta, pizza, kulcha, bhatura, etc. that are so tempting, should be avoided as much as possible. You can have these twice a week and only on days that you exercise.
- Avoid black colas as they decay your bones and internal organs.
- Make sure your broccoli, watermelon, bhindi, etc., are not coloured green. Wash your vegetables really well before cooking.

flax seeds every day. And the good part about it is that you don't need to worry about buying it every day; just keep it in a small ziplock or in a box with a spoon. You can even carry it easily in your purse while travelling or anywhere you go. Isn't this uncomplicated and simple?

Flax seeds contain omega 3 fatty acids, which are not found naturally in the body. As a result, we need to supplement it in our body from outside. Omega 3 fatty acids are commonly found in flax seeds, fishes; like tuna and sardines, soyabean, tofu, spinach, cauliflower, broccoli, pumpkin seeds, etc. It is also found in dry fruits, and nuts especially walnuts.

How is omega 3 fatty acid useful in preventing ageing? Omega 3 fatty acid is beneficial to the body in numerous ways. First, it prevents any kinds of fatigue and depression, keeping you active and lively most of the times. It works on your mind and your moods, and hence is also highly recommended during periods or during PMS. It is also extremely useful in controlling the excessive white discharge in women that many find annoying and embarrassing. Second, it keeps your skin soft and supple and prevents wrinkling; makes your hair thick and shiny and can delay greying; keeps your nails strong and prevents yellowing; and is beneficial during migraines.

Third, it is wonderful for the joints. All nagging joint pains, which are one of the most prominent signs of ageing, can be taken care of by having flax seeds. Last, it helps in keeping your heart healthy by reducing the cholesterol levels in the blood. Hence, you have less chances of being inflicted with hypertension, high blood pressure, clogged arteries, etc.

Be your own beautician

Early and excessive use of make-up is extremely harmful for the body, especially your skin. These days, young school girls in their pre-teens start using cosmetics meant for adults. Sadly, their mothers not only allow them to use make-up but also encourage them, thinking it is a girly thing and will make them look prettier. But in reality, they are just spoiling their daughters' skin, which will make them look older than other girls their age.

In India, there is a fascination for looking as fair as possible. Sadly, our obsession for white skin is still not over. It is not spoken aloud openly just to be politically correct. The matrimonial ads are full of 'looking for milky white brides' and hence parents feel that the fairer their daughter is, the better her chances of finding a good groom. So they end up going for skin lightening, bleaching the skin, etc. What they don't realize is that these contain strong chemicals, which do irreparable damage to the skin.

If you are in the service industry, media, or films, etc., and your line of work demands that you use make-up regularly, you should make sure that you do not sleep with make-up on and clean your skin before sleeping. Also, use good products, which do not harm your skin.

Principle 3: Have sex at least 3 times a week

Rahul Verma, 32, had a girlfriend but broke up with her one and a half years back. Since then, he hasn't got another girlfriend though he is addicted to online dating. He chats for hours on the internet, and doesn't like to go out much with his friends. Rahul gets irritated and angry very easily nowadays and as he leads mostly sedentary lifestyle. His stomach has turned flabby. He has also been experiencing gradual hair fall, but he doesn't care much about it. He now looks like an older and angrier version of the once hip and cheerful Rahul. His friends barely recognize him, but Rahul couldn't care less as he his happy with the friends he has made on the internet.

And this brings me to my third rule for looking young, which is to have sex at least three times a week. Few people know and acknowledge the benefits of sex for a healthy and youthful life. And it is high time we give sex its due credit. Sex is the natural rhythm of life. Whenever you have sex, you not only burn 450 calories, but your body releases hormones that keep your mind calm and your body flexible. It is very important for staying young and active. A healthy sex life is also a prerequisite for a good marriage or relationship. It is something special that you share with your partner, and what is best is that it makes you look younger.

Mallika Mehta is 35, and divorced with a handicapped son. She is a successful businesswoman, with her own construction company. After her divorce, Mallika tried to keep herself happy, and started learning Salsa. She is very happy with her professional life and has an affluent lifestyle with three houses in Mumbai. She tried dating again after a long break, and even tried the online marriage portals but nothing seemed to work out as most of the men she found were more interested in her money than her. Today Mallika gyms regularly, and treats herself to the best of holidays, but feels depressed and lonely most of the time as she is not able to find a suitable partner for herself. She has almost given up hope now, and has started looking older. One of the reasons for this, I feel, is the lack of love and sex in her life.

Many women after having children or as they grow older start ignoring the needs of their own body. Remember it is never too late to have sex. It is a basic requirement of your body like food and water, and there is nothing embarrassing about having sexual desires. Sex is a natural desire of the body, and this is the way God has created us. There is no point denying sex to yourself and your partner.

Principle 4: Do any physical activity at least three times a week

Through my fourth principle, I want to stress on the importance of physical activity for staying and looking young. You must take up some form of physical activity, depending on your age, at least three times a week. It does not matter how old you are: there is always something you can do. Remember, the more you exert, the more fit and flexible you will be. The inverted postures in yoga are extremely good for preventing ageing. When you do such inverted postures, the blood flow gets directed to the particular organ, and the oxygen supply to that part increases. The most popular postures which help in rejuvenation are Sarvangasana, Poornhalasana, Matsyasana, etc. However, these postures should be performed only under expert guidance.

Ankita Sehgal is a 28-year-old woman working for an insurance company. She is married, with a son, and lives on the seventh floor of her apartment building. Although Ankita does not exercise regularly, she makes it a point never to take the lift and climbs up the stairs instead, unless she has something really heavy to carry. She also walks to her workplace, which is three kilometres away. No wonder Ankita is slim and fit without any regular workout. So you see, you don't always need to go to the gym or do yoga to stay young and fit. Little changes in your lifestyle can also make a difference.

Women in their twenties can do anything from yoga, gym, aerobics, dancing, walking, jogging, running, to all kinds of sports, especially swimming and cycling. When you are in your twenties, your body is flexible and can easily adapt to any kind of physical activity. Do what you like the most but do it at least three times a week.

Women in their thirties can also do most of the things that a twenty year old can like yoga, gym, aerobics, dancing, walking, cycling, etc. However, you cannot jog or run as well, or as fast, as you used to do when you were in your teens or your twenties. Also, you can play only those sports that you started when you were young. You should not take up a completely new sport in your thirties as it can over strain and damage your body.

When you are in your forties your choices get even more limited but there are still many things that you can do. You can of course do yoga as there is no age to begin yoga, and you can do it at any point of your life. Go to the gym only if you have been gymming regularly, and don't start a new sport. You can do swimming, and cycling if your joints are fine, and do not give you much trouble. You may also continue playing a sport you started when you were young, and that to which your body is already acclimatized. Sridevi plays tennis with her daughters and does yoga regularly. Here's what her exercise routine is like.

Sridevi's exercise routine

Age: 40 plus   **Weight:** 56 kilos   **Sessions:** 1½ hour; six days a week

Target: Initially her goal was to lose weight but now it is to maintain it, and keep her body toned. These exercises improve blood circulation, keep her sinusitis problem in check and are also good for looking young, improving flexibility, and feeling energetic. On Friday and Saturday, Sridevi does cardio activities like playing badminton or walking on the treadmill.

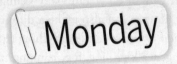

Monday

Monday's workout is all about rejuvenation and feeling energetic.

1. We start our day with a light warm up, then she runs on a treadmill for at least 10 minutes.
2. After 5 minutes of relaxation we do some postures for flexibility like Virasana, Trikonasana, Vakrasana for at least 30 minutes.
3. Lastly we do about 25 Suryanamaskars.
4. After 5 minutes of relaxation, do Pranayam along Kapalbhati for around 10 to 15 minutes.

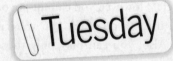

Tuesday

On Tuesday, we concentrate on the abdomen.

1. We start with 200 strokes of Kapalbhati (to remove the toxins in the body).
2. This is followed by light warm up exercises to open up the body muscles and joints.
3. We do 20 normal and 10 slow Suryanamaskars and then relaxation of 5 minutes.
4. We do variations of Suryanamaskars including cardio (to increase the metabolic rate of your body) like running for 1 minute and 2 Suryanamaskars for 5 rounds.
5. A relaxation break for 5 minutes follows.
6. We do different postures for the stomach to achieve a flat stomach—like Ardha Halasana with hands behind the neck for support and then raising the shoulders up, for 20 seconds and moving the upper body 20 to 25 times.
7. Triyak Naukasana: When in Naukasana, turn your body just a little towards your right side, holding the same position and gently moving back and forth. Repeat it with the other side. Do this for around 30 minutes. When working on abs, normally one gets a backache. So it is very important to do counter poses like in this case, Ardha Setubandhasana or Chakrasana along with twisting on the floor. By doing this your neck tends to get stiff so follow up with 3 sets of neck rotations in clockwise and anticlockwise directions.
8. Finish with 200 strokes of Kapalbhatis alongwith 5 rounds of Anulom Vilom.

{ My message to my fans is to think healthy, eat healthy, avoid junk food, and practise yoga with Payal. }

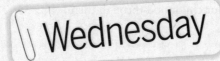

Wednesday

Wednesdays' workout is all about the lower body, that is, legs, butt, and outer thighs.

1 Normal stretches for warm up: 5–6 minutes
2 Spot jogging: 10 minutes
3 Suryanamaskar with variations: Keep your left and right legs forward just like in position 4 and 9 of Suryanamaskar. We do it 10 times with each leg. This helps to tone your hip muscles, quadriceps, and inner thighs.
4 For quadriceps we do the chair pose, holding it for 30 seconds. Repeat it 20 times, 5 rounds

5 For outer thighs, move sideways with one leg going up and down with the upper body remaining straight: 30 to 50 times

Stretching positions for each muscle worked on:

1 Paschimottanasana for hamstrings: 15 seconds, 2 sets
2 Dhanurasana for quadriceps: 15 seconds, 2 sets
3 Ardha Kapotasana for outer thighs and butt: 15 seconds, right and left side, 1 set
4 End up with Bhastrika and Om chanting.

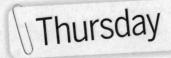

Thursday

Thursdays are for sides and obliques. We do Suryanamaskars on all six days because this is the only way you can use all your muscles

1 Running: 20 minutes
2 Simple static and dynamic stretching exercises
3 Suryanamaskar: 25 rounds, 2 sets
4 Sideways Naukasana: Lie down sideways on your right. Slowly lift both your legs and hold it there for 10 seconds. Bring your legs up and down 20 times and hold it again for

10 seconds. Do 5 rounds each on both sides. Similarly, do this with your upper and lower body as well. The only difference is that the up and down movement in this case would be 30 times.

Standing positions:

1. Side bending Chakrasana: 2 sets
2. Tadasana: 2 sets
3. Parighasana: 2 sets
4. End with 5 rounds of Bhastrika and 5 rounds of Bhramari Pranayam

When you cross 50, the best things to do are yoga, meditation, relaxation, and regular walks. Don't be a couch potato—watching TV, and cribbing about your problems. Instead, be active and take an interest in your grandchildren and relive your childhood through them.

Physical activity ideas for women who are thirty-plus

- Take the stairs up not the elevator
- Go buy your own groceries
- Park your car a little away from your destination
- Cycle it out
- Walk your pet yourself
- Walk in your park
- Answer your doorbell yourself
- Keep your tea cups in the kitchen yourself
- Walk and go to the pantry
- Keep only one glass of water not a bottle; so that you get up to get another glass

Principle 5: Be childlike and creative

Have you noticed how most artists, painters, and dancers, look younger than their age? Their secret lies in my fifth principle for being young. You must encourage the child inside you and undertake creative pursuits that give you happiness and satisfaction. Artists often live in their own worlds, and relish their connection to art and creativity. When they create anything new or practise what they love, it gives them immense pleasure, which releases youth hormones in the body that circulate in the blood, and fight diseases and old age. Out of this state of contentment and bliss, comes the elixir of youth.

I cannot find a better example than Sridevi to illustrate this point. Sridevi has been painting since she was a child but had left it due to her busy career. And when she got married, she got totally engrossed in her kids. But now that her kids are a little older, she has started painting again. Painting is such a creative process and she gets immense satisfaction from it. She can put her thoughts on to the canvas and to play with colours. Recently, when her painting was auctioned for charity, she felt touched that she could help others with what was a hobby for her. She also plays tennis with her children, and the combination of mental and physical activity is the secret of her timeless beauty.

So go back to your childhood, and do things that you enjoyed the most; be it painting, dancing, pottery if you enjoyed playing with mud, etc. Don't be scared to be curious or ask questions. Forget your daily troubles, and take out time to pursue things in which you find contentment. It's no secret that all grandparents love playing and spending time with their grand children. So live your childhood through your grandchildren. Walk with them, play with them and laugh with them. Play on; it's still fun and it'll keep you young.

Also, get adventurous in life and do things that you have never done before. An adventure, by nature, is embarking on a journey where you don't know what is going to happen next. It involves discovering and learning from everything around you and every moment that passes by. The unpredictabililty is actually fun. Mountaineering, trekking, hiking, travelling to

Creative things to do at any age

- Pottery
- Painting
- Dancing
- Singing
- Writing
- Playing an instrument
- Redecorating/redoing your house
- Trying out new recipes, new cuisines
- Playing with or looking after pets if you are an animal lover

small places, skydiving, bungee jumping, etc., are all examples of such activities. However, you should choose these activities based on your health and fitness levels.

Most of the times, we are so busy in our daily routine that we don't have the time for anything else. We just surrender to life and look forward to what life is going to offer next. We are ready for anything and accept everything that it gives. Getting adventurous, I think, forms an important ingredient of fitness. Enjoying yoga, the asanas and pranayam, gives you more benefits than when you just do it mechanically.

Nature is something that has been given to us in abundance, without any cost or conditions. Simple everyday things like observing rain, watching the moonlight, or being around greenery makes us feel fresher and more energetic. The harmony and balance of nature is actually the best teacher that one could get. Nature gives without asking and is always there for us. As an integral part of nature, we too were born with harmonious and balanced bodies, and we should go back to nature to reclaim it to look and feel younger.

Principle 6: Use the dustbin for bad memories

My sixth and last principle for looking ten years younger relates to your mental state. Always discard as many bad memories, things, incidents that you can. You must never carry more baggage than is absolutely necessary. Don't get me wrong. This does not mean that you should not worry about your family, job, career, relationships, etc. What I mean is that there are many things that are not so important and we shouldn't worry about them—like what's happening in the TV soaps, what your neighbours bought for Diwali, how many cars your friend has, etc. You can surely live without worrying yourself sick about these things.

Ayesha Khan is 36 and had a baby just four months back. A new mother, she has taken a break from her job in an MNC to concentrate on her baby. Ayesha was used to an active life but since her baby was born, she feels her life has totally changed. She can hardly go out and finds managing things very difficult. Her husband has a busy travelling job and is out most of the time. She is getting increasingly frustrated with each passing day and has stopped taking care of herself. As a result, she's not able to lose her pregnancy weight, and this has made her even more irritated and restless. The couple are embroiled in regular fights now over minor issues, which they would overlook earlier.

You must also avoid all unpleasant things and situations like fights, arguments, and tiffs. Don't pick fights unnecessarily to vent your day-to-day frustration. We are lucky to be living in a world where couples are increasingly getting aware of their rights. Nobody is perfect and we should all remember that. Although it is normal to fight, we should not make it a habit and pester each other unnecessarily or make unreasonable demands. You might not realize it, but in dominating your partner or creating a fight, you are harming your own body. You will age faster, and no amount of money or branded products will be able to bring back your youth. Remember equality is important but keep jealousy at bay. Don't carry any grudge: finish it off then and there, and chuck it in the dustbin. Always keep this imaginary dustbin next to you, and throw away all unwanted emotions and things.

Never habour any ill-feeling against others. Solve, resolve, and move forward in life. Let go of things. Forgiveness not only helps others but is also good for you. Move with the flow—live in the present not in the past or your future. This will, believe me, help you stay at least ten years younger. The inner contentment and peace will reflect in your skin, hair, face, and all your body parts.

Yoga to fight ageing

What is the thing that most of us are scared of as we grow older? With every birthday cake that we cut, with every year that trickles by noiselessly what worries us most is ageing. And the most prominent sign of ageing is the wrinkle; the tell-tale lines on the face. Sagging skin and loss of elasticity results in wrinkles on the body, and the face. Another apparent indication of ageing is greying hair. But luckily, yoga has remedies for wrinkles as well as greying hair. I'm not saying that by doing yoga you will never have wrinkles, or that your hair will never turn grey, but you can certainly delay them and prevent premature ageing that is becoming so common nowadays. Earlier these marks would appear in the forties, now it can be commonly seen in people in their thirties or even twenties.

For the face

Kriyas such as Kapalbhati and Jalneti are extremely good for the face. Kapal means 'head' while bhati means 'glow'. Jalneti increases the blood flow in the face and opens up the blockages of nostrils to enable us to inhale properly. Breathing properly is very important to get more oxygen into the body. Asanas, especially inverted postures like Vipreetkarni, Poorna Halasana, and Shirshasana direct the blood flow towards the head. Simhasana helps stretch the facial muscles, and keep them firm and elastic. Pranayam, like Anulom Vilom cleanses

Workout for your face only

Probably the first thing that we look at when we meet anybody is their face. And one of the many things that instantly strike us, consciously or unconsciously, is their age as reflected on their face. However, healthy and taut (free of wrinkles) facial skin can keep people from guessing your age. Below is a list of specific exercises that you can do to control wrinkles and dark circles and keep your skin firm:

- Trataka: 25 seconds to begin with but you should keep increasing the time slowly and gradually
- Jalneti kriya: 3 times a week

veins and asteries, helping you breathe better and, keeping your face fresh and toned.

For the neck

Ageing shows clearly on your neck, and sometimes we're so busy concentrating on our face that we ignore our neck completely. Asanas like Matyasana reduce the fat from the back of your neck. When you do Brahma Mudra by turning your neck towards right, left, upwards, and downwards to twist and stretch the neck muscles, it improves the elasticity of the skin and muscles on the neck.

For the hair

We Indians are blessed with luscious black hair, which is a hallmark of our beauty. After your skin, it is your hair which makes you stand out in a crowd. Healthy hair is a sign of a healthy body. But nowadays not many are able to bask in

Workout for your neck only

All of us have different problem areas—some of us are prone to dark circles while some may have loose skin on the neck. The set of exercises given below specially targets the skin of your neck, where ageing shows unmistakably, and helps to keep it taut and firm. You can do these six days in a week.
Duration: 15 minutes

- Brahma Mudra: 5 rounds
- Ustrasana: hold for 20 seconds, 2 sets
- Niralambasana: hold for 30 seconds, 2 sets

the glory of a lovely dark mane for long, what with ageing catching up sooner than expected. Mitali Jain, a 28-year-old event manager, got really worried as her hair had already started greying. She just could not understand why this was happening to her. Her mother's hair was still salt and pepper, and had started turning grey only after she had crossed 40. There are many Mitalis out there who are facing such a situation today due to our dietary, lifestyle, and health changes. What can you do if you are one of them? All the following exercises especially the inverted postures improve the strength of the hair and stop greying as they act on the upper extremity of the body. Below is a workout specially designed for people who want to have dark healthy hair for as long as possible.

Workout to prevent wrinkles and greying of hair

I would now like to share with you a basic workout that I have designed to stay young. These sets of asanas, if done regularly, control wrinkles on the face and the neck and keep your hair black. You need to do this routine three days in a week.

Basic precautions

1. Never workout on a heavy stomach.
2. Exercise preferably two hours after your breakfast and four hours after your lunch.
3. Drink at least 4 to 5 litres of water in a day to avoid constipation and indigestion.
4. There should be a break of at least 10 seconds between each asana in the sequence.

5. If you have any kind of ailment or health related issues please consult your doctor before doing any exercise or do it under the guidance of a yoga teacher.

Where: Choose a place which has fresh air circulation preferably a garden, a terrace, or a workout place in your house.

What you need: A yoga mat, Jalneti pot, and a hand or a face towel.

1. You need to start by performing Jalneti. To prepare for Jalneti, place the mat on the floor, and sit in any comfortable position on the mat. Start with breathing 5 times with focus. After this, close your right nostril with your right thumb and inhale and exhale with the right nostil 5 times. Now remove the thumb from the right nostril and close the left nostril with the middle and index finger of your right hand. Inhale and exhale with the right nostril 5 times to open up and clean your nostrils.

   Now you are ready to perform Jalneti. You need to be near a wash basin or someplace where you brush your teeth when you do this kriya. Add a pinch of salt in a glass of lukewarm water and mix it properly. Transfer the water to the Jalneti pot, bend forward in a 90-degree angle to the floor, then turn your neck towards the left side and open your mouth to inhale and exhale. Now with the Jalneti pipe, let the water enter your left nostril and allow it to come through the other nostril while breathing from the mouth. Continue to do this till the Jalneti pot is empty. After you have completed this process, do 30 strokes of Kapalbhati, in standing position, facing the wash basin, to clean your nostril. Perform the same procedure with the other nostril.

   There are many benefits of Jalneti. It opens up blockages

in the nose and in the blood vessels in the face, thereby allowing a better flow of blood and oxygen to the facial muscles.

2. After the Jalneti kriya, sit again on your yoga mat on the floor and do 50 strokes of Kapalbhati in 2 rounds.

3. Now relax in Shavasana for 5 minutes to rest your facial muscles.

4. We now begin with the asanas. The first one is Vipreetkarni in supine position. Put your feet together and your hands by the sides with palms resting on the floor. Now inhale slowly and while exhaling raise both your legs up 90 degrees to the floor, then push your palms on the floor, and raise your hips up. Hold your waist with your hands in the final position. Remember to keep your neck muscles relaxed and to breathe normally. Stay in this position for 15 to 20 seconds, then slowly come back to the original position. Follow it up with its counter pose Setubandhasana.

   Vipreetkarni is extremely good as it directs and increases the blood flow towards the head. Regular practise of this asana keeps your heart, brain and facial muscles young forever.

5. Poorna Halasana: Just as with Vipreetkarni, try to raise your legs upwards towards your head in a 180-degree angle and hold it for 15 seconds. Breathe normally and keep your muscles relaxed. Now come back to the original position in the reverse manner. This is an advanced asana and has benefits similar to Vipreetkarni, like massaging the internal organs of the body. Remember to do its counterpose Kati Chakrasana for 15 seconds on each side. Relax for 2 minutes.

6. Simhasana: To begin Simhasana, first sit in Vajrasana on your knees and place your palms on your knees, making sure that your elbows are straight. Now inhale slowly and while exhaling stretch your facial muscles by pulling out your tongue and pressing it downwards towards the chin. While you are doing this, make sure that you look between your eyebrows. Hold it for 15 to 20 seconds, while breathing normally. Repeat it 3 to 5 times.

7. Matsyasana: Sit in Padmasana. Now taking the help of your elbow, slowly bend backwards and lie on your back. Next, raise your head with the help of your hands and place the upper part of your head on the floor, pulling the chin upwards. Hold your toes with your index finger and keep the elbows on the ground at the same time. Hold it like this for 15 seconds, before you come back to the original position. Do it for 2 rounds.

    Matsyasana or the fish pose is supposed to be good for many health related problems. When you are doing this asana, you apply pressure on your neck, abdomen and even pelvic areas. Hence, it is good for the nervous system, kidneys, stomach, intestines, and the pelvic organs and makes them strong.

8. Brahma Mudra: Sit in Padmasana in Gyan Mudra. Now slowly turn your neck towards the right and stay there for 5 seconds, then repeat the process with the other side and hold again for 5 seconds. Now bring your neck back to the original position and raise your chin up. Hold for 5 seconds, then slowly bring your neck down and come back to the original position.

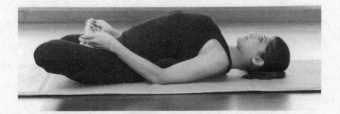

Saral Matsyasana

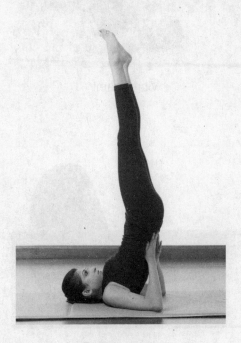

Sarvangasana

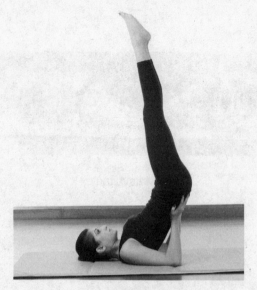

Vipreetkarni

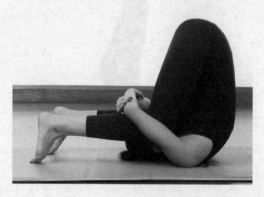

Karnapidasana

6

The real secret of beauty

I was really lucky to find Payal, and that too so early on in my film career. Being Miss Sri Lanka, I was already conscious about my looks, but what Payal taught me was how to maintain them, and improve. So what does beauty mean to me? According to me, a glowing skin is the most important aspect of beauty. If you have good skin, half your worries are taken care of. Next on my list is healthy shiny hair. When I first came to Mumbai, I took some time to get used to the humidity and my hectic schedule. I realized I had to be disciplined and follow my beauty routines diligently. Like all other film stars, I too have a tough lifestyle. We have to travel a lot, work long hours, sometimes in the sun, and even put on heavy make up almost every day. I was really worried how to do all this and yet stay beautiful. Believe me, it's not so easy to be a star and look like one all the time.

I am especially conscious of taking care of my skin, as I feel that it is the most important aspect of beauty. There are so many small things that we disregard in daily life. Like do you know how important sweating is for the skin? When we exercise and sweat, the pores of the body open up and the toxins are thrown out of the body. After each session of exercise, I feel as if my body has come alive, and my skin has started breathing, feeling soft and nourished. One of the other things I do is to remove all make-up as soon as the shoot is over, and moisturize my skin. I also wear sunglasses whenever I go out to protect my eyes from the sun, dust, and pollution. It's not only a style statement! If you want to look fresh and beautiful like me, take care of yourself and exercise regularly.

Jackie

Jacqueline

In this chapter, let's look at things we can do to look more beautiful by taking care of our skin, hair, and eyes.

I am not going to delve into the intricacies of what our body is made up of, how it functions and stays healthy, as I am no beauty expert. But what I will do in the following pages is share with you my experiences, what I do to take care of myself, and what I've learnt from my mother who is a beauty expert. There are also specific yoga exercises for beauty, which I will talk about in detail in this chapter. Our Bollywood beauties too will share with you their own beauty regimes and tips that make them looking stunning and photo ready always.

Who doesn't want to look beautiful? All of us dream of looking attractive, and wish we could resemble our favourite stars. Like me you too must have wished at some point or the other to look like Kareena, Katrina, Aishwarya, Rani, or Jacqueline. Nothing gives a better high than somebody complimenting, 'Oh, you look like Kareena' or 'Your skin glows like Jacqueline's'. In India, stars are our benchmark for beauty. We vie for their great bodies, glowing skin, lustrous hair, and clear sparkling eyes. I recently read an article on cosmetic surgery in the newspaper that said how

scores of women were approaching doctors saying that they
want Aishwarya's jawline, her aquiline nose, and even her
eyebrows. Some others wanted to have Kareena's flawless
skin and Katrina's pouty lips. But you don't always have to
undergo surgery to look beautiful. You can make the best of
your own assets and look beautiful in your own right without
going under the knife.

Not all stars are born with perfect bodies and flawless skin.
They work on their beauty and take care of themselves to look
the way they do. And then to maintain it is even trickier. You
will know what I mean if you remember Rekha in *Saawan
Bhado,* or more recently Shilpa Shetty in *Baazigar*. Both of
them have undergone quite a transformation since the time
they first started out in Bollywood. Rekha is the epitome of
beauty even at 55, while Shilpa has never looked better than
what she does now. They have worked hard to look the way
they do today.

According to me, the most important aspects of beauty are
a perfect ten body (that we talked about in chapter two), a
clear and supple skin, radiant hair (yes, it is very important!),
and bright eyes. These are the four basic areas that you need
to focus on. You might not have the perfect face, but if you
have a lovely body, skin, hair, and eyes, there is no doubt that
you will make heads turn. Believe me, you will be noticed, just
like the stars.

Skin care

My school friend Prerna Kapoor was undoubtedly the
prettiest girl in our class. She was slim, had a lovely figure,
was blessed with cream and peaches skin, and the boys

adored her completely. Since we passed out of school, we both got engrossed in our own lives and lost touch with each other. Recently, I bumped into her at a friend's house and was surprised to find her a distant image of her old self. Prerna, now 35, is a financial analyst with an MNC. Although she is still slim with a toned body, she had glaring dark circles under her eyes, which dominated her face.

I strongly believe that beauty begins with a beautiful skin. Many people say that your eyes are a reflection of your mind and what you are thinking, but I believe that the skin can talk as well. Your past, habits, lifestyle, etc., can all be determined looking at your skin. Believe me, it's possible! A healthy glowing skin is a reflection of the internal health of your body while a prematurely wrinkled, scarred, or dull skin reflects the neglect that it has gone through in terms of skin care, diet, sleep, bad habits, etc. The markets today are flooded with countless beauty products of all kinds. Their attractive packaging and catchy marketing campaigns often tempt us into buying them and trying them out at least once. Who would not like to be 'fairer in 15 days' or 'have pimple-free skin in 3 days'? Whatever I buy, I make sure that it has as little chemicals as possible, because in the long run chemicals can severely damage your skin. Always go for organic, natural, or even home-based beauty products with minimal chemicals.

The skin is the outer exposed covering of our body. It is what takes the brunt of everything first, be it harsh weather, sunlight, smoke, dust, pollution, or anything else in the atmosphere. The skin is made up of tissues and cells just like other parts of our body, and it too needs to breathe. It gets oxygen through the bloodstream that circulates inside our body and protects the delicate organs inside, also playing a significant role in disposing off waste materials out of our system through its numerous pores.

Our skin can be dry, normal, oily, or a combination of all these. You can do a simple test at home to find out what skin type you are. When you wake up in the morning, if your skin is shiny throughout, you have oily skin. If on the other hand, your skin feels stretched, as if it is being pulled from the sides, it is dry. Some people might have shiny skin only on the T zone (forehead, nose, and chin) while feeling stretched on the rest of the face. Such people have combination skin. If your skin does not have any of these characteristics in the morning when you wake up, it means you have normal skin.

Since the skin is the exposed part of our body, ageing shows first on our skin. There are some simple basic things in our daily life that we ignore or are unaware of, but which make a huge difference to our skin. You might have noticed the hands of housewives who wash clothes. The skin, especially of the fingers and the hand, becomes thin and wrinkled as a result of being exposed to harsh chemicals found in the detergents on a regular basis. Did you know that there's a way you can avoid this? Yes, and it's simple and uncomplicated. First, avoid dipping your hands in the water to soak the clothes. Use a small stick or even an old toothbrush. Second, make sure that you moisturize your skin before and after washing clothes. If you follow this practice diligently, you can protect the skin of your hand, from sagging or getting wrinkled prematurely.

Most men have really rough facial skin and beard like copper wires. Men too need to take care of their skin! For smooth facial skin you must not use foams for shaving.

Instead use a cream and massage the cream into your skin for at least 10 minutes before your shave. This will keep your skin soft and supple. Finish off with a good aftershave lotion every time you use a razor on your face.

Yoga brought a glow to my complexion

My tryst with yoga began about seven years ago when my friend recommended Power Yoga to me as a complete workout. I tried my hand at it but gravitated back to my traditional workout that combined cardio and weight training exercises. But about two or three years ago—and this coincided with my preparation for *Dil Bole Hadippa*—I began looking for a change in my exercise regime. It was around this time that I met Payal who helped me gradually include yoga in my life. What started out as a means to get fitter and get my body toned, has now become a way of life for me.

I began to divide my time equally between cardio and weight training on one hand, and yoga on the other. But slowly, over the last seven or eight months, I've moved on to four days a week of only yoga. Although fitness and toning my body were the primary aims, I soon began to notice visible changes in the way I felt and looked, in addition to better stamina and improvement in my fitness levels. I learned that a lot of the postures or asanas were working on my body from the inside. Yoga combines cardio, stretches, and rhythmic breathing that helps the body rid itself of any toxins or blockages thereby increasing blood circulation. This is what I feel has brought a glow to my complexion.

Much has been written about my lean look in *Dil Bole*

Hadippa, but I would like to affirm that I have never deprived myself of any kind of food. I've often noticed that men increase their protein intake and cut down on carbohydrates to build muscle, and sometimes, women are also asked to do the same. But in my opinion this is detrimental as an unbalanced diet can make them look aged in addition to making them irritable. My effort was purely to get fitter and I didn't want my skin to get affected or look haggard. I also didn't see the point in depriving my body of food that I was accustomed to since childhood. I felt that this could lead to binge eating, cravings and withdrawal pangs.

It is because of yoga that I feel in tune with my body and am completely aware of the foods that are good and nutritious, and tend to keep away from anything that is unhealthy. It's almost as though now my body rejects anything that can cause harm.

For me, beauty has never just been skin-deep and it's not just about the expensive skincare and make up products that are used externally. You will notice that the most beautiful people are often those who feel good about themselves and are happy with themselves. Yoga is a major contributor to helping me maintain an inner equilibrium. Of course, it is very important to look into external factors that act upon the skin. I am very particular about scrubbing my skin clean of make-up as soon as a shoot wraps up. A good skin care regime, healthy diet, and yoga, I feel, are the inseparable factors that contribute towards a healthy skin.

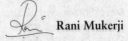 **Rani Mukerji**

Rani Mukerji's exercise routine

Age: 30 plus **Sessions:** 1 hour; 3 days a week
Target: To stay fit and look good.
Besides the exercises below, we do 100 Suryanamaskars the days Rani does not feel tired. We also do Shank Prakshalana on days we want to cleanse the entire digestive tract.

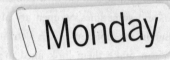

Monday

1. Climbing stairs for 30 minutes
2. 10 Suryanamaskars + kicking forward with each leg, 50 seconds
3. 10 Suryanamaskars + kicking sideways with each leg, 50 seconds
4. 10 Suryanamaskars + kicking backwards with each leg, 50 seconds
5. 20 regular Suryanamaskars

Standing positions:

6. Parvatasana: hold for 20 seconds, each leg, 3 sets
7. Utkatasana: hold for 20 seconds, 3 sets

Prone positions:

8. Ardha Shalabhasana: hold for 20 seconds, each side, 2 sets
9. Poorna Shalabhasana: hold for 20 seconds, 2 sets

Sitting positions:

10. Supta Vajrasana: hold for 20 seconds, 2 sets
11. Sharnagat Mudra: hold for 20 seconds
12. Shavasana: 2 minutes
13. Kapalbhati: 250 strokes, 4 sets
14. Anulom Vilom Pranayam: 5 rounds
15. Om chanting: 5 rounds

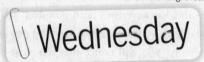

Wednesday

1. Warm up for 5 minutes
2. 10 regular Suryanamaskars
3. 1 Suryanamaskar with 50 kapalbhatis while standing, 10 rounds
4. 1 Suryanamaskar with 5 push ups (in position 5 of Suryanamaskar), 10 sets
5. 1 Suryanamaskar with 30 lunges, 10 rounds

Prone positions:

6. Cat pose with elbow bent: hold for 20 seconds, 5 sets
7. Get into Bhujangasana to do Sarpasana: hold for 10 seconds, 10 sets
8. Chakrasana standing sideways with the feet apart: hold for 10 seconds, each side, 5 sets
9. Chakrasana standing sideways with the feet together: hold for 10 seconds, each side, 5 sets

Standing positions:

10. Triyak Bhujangasana on the stomach: 10 seconds, each side, 3 times

Supine positions:

11. Kati Chakrasana on the back: 10 seconds, each side, 3 times
12. Relax in Shavasana: 2 minutes
13. Bhastrika Pranayam: 5 rounds, 20 strokes of Kapalbhati + 1 round Anulom Vilom= 1 Bhastrika Pranayam
14. Sit in Vajrasana for 2 minutes with eyes closed

> { While I'm very particular about my work out, I believe in giving my body enough rest and never obsess about the days I skip a workout. }

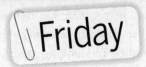

Friday

1. Warm up: 5 minutes
2. 25 Suryanamaskars, 2 sets
3. Spot jogging for 15 seconds + 50 Kapalbhati strokes, 5 sets
4. Ek Pada Janu Shirshasana: hold for 15 seconds, each side, 3 sets
5. Natrajasana: hold for 10 seconds, each leg, 3 sets
6. Ardha Chandrasana while standing: hold for 10 seconds, each side, 3 sets
7. Naukasana on the back: hold for 10 seconds, 2 sets
8. Chakrasana: hold for 10 seconds, 2 sets
9. Poorna Halasana: hold for 10 seconds, 2 sets
10. Setubandhasana: hold for 10 seconds, 2 sets
11. Dhanurasana on the stomach: hold for 10 seconds, 2 sets
12. Naukasana on the stomach: hold for 10 seconds, 2 sets
13. Matsyendrasana: hold for 10 seconds, each side, 2 sets
14. Parvatasana in Padmasana: hold for 10 seconds, 2 sets
15. Relax in Shavasana: 5 minutes
16. Sheetali Prayanam: 5 rounds
17. End with Om chanting: 5 rounds

A beauty routine is a must

Amrita Sachdeva, a 24-year-old model has been smoking since the age of 16. She would put on make-up and shoot outdoors, sometimes in the sun for hours. Often Amrita would not remove her make-up after her shoots. Very soon, her skin started wrinkling and looking papery. Now at 25, she has the skin of a 35-year-old!

A few of you might be thinking: how do I start taking care of my skin? The first and foremost thing is to follow a beauty routine. Most of you will be surprised if I told you that Kareena has never done a single facial in her life. But she is genetically blessed, and what she does instead is lead a disciplined lifestyle with a basic beauty routine, which keeps her glowing always. In fact, Kareena looks gorgeous even without make-up as her skin does all the talking.

Why do we need a routine at all? We are all creatures of habit. I am now so used to cleaning my face and removing all make-up before I go to bed that I cannot sleep without doing that. Even though I might be really exhausted after a late-night party or a family function, I have to remove my make-up before I sleep. But my reward is my fresh and happy skin when I wake up the next morning. So if you inculcate a good habit early on, you will reap its benefits throughout your life. You will take care of yourself as a habit and not out of compulsion. In fact, if you follow a beauty routine regularly, there is not much else you need to do to look beautiful. Many of us in our early to late twenties or early thirties, suddenly wake up to the realization one fine day that our skin is not as taut as it used to be, or not as clear as it was in our teens; that there are dark spots and fine lines on our face around our eyes; our hair has become dull and started greying; and our nails look yellow and brittle. Did this happen overnight? No, not at all! This is just the result of years of ignoring our body. So wake up before it is too late. Nowadays, you must consciously start taking care of your skin from the time you hit the early twenties. In fact, the sooner you start following a beauty routine, the better it is for you.

The three basic steps that everybody needs to follow irrespective of their skin type is: cleaning, toning, moisturizing. Here's a simple beauty routine that I follow which really works for me:

Morning after waking up
1. I wash my face with an organic facewash suited to my skin type with cold water.
2. I then apply a toner followed by a moisturizer with an SPF of at least 15.

Afternoon/lunch time
1. I try and wash my face once during lunch time, and then reapply the moisturizer.

Evening
1. After my work for the day is over and I come back home, I wash my face again and reapply the moisturizer in the evening. On days when I am working late or get back home only in the night, I usually skip this step. However, if you have oily skin, spend most of the day outdoors, or have to wear heavy make-up, then you should try and wash your face in the evenings too.

Night

1. Before I sleep, as I mentioned, I make sure that I clean my face, and take off all make-up.
2. I then mix two drops of moisturizer with two drops of water and apply it on my face. I leave it on for sometime, but before I go to bed, I wipe my face with a tissue to remove any excess oil.
3. And, of course, I take care to leave the area under my eyes bare as it does not need any moisturizing or massaging.

So as you would have noticed in my routine, I need to wash my face at least three times a day under normal circumstances. You might need to do it more often if you are travelling, are out most of the day, have put on heavy make-up, or if you have oily skin. People with oily skin should wash their face at least four to five times in a day to avoid acnes and pimples. Skin-care routines are just like brushing our teeth; once we make it a habit, it will happen automatically.

Use as little make-up as you can

Whenever I think about ageing I automatically think of my mother Jyoti Gidwani. I wish I could age as gracefully as her. She has never coloured her hair or bleached her skin, and has a lovely salt and pepper crop now. My mother is 57 years old. And believe me, her skin is that of a 35-year-old with not a single line or wrinkle on her face. While I was growing up, most people thought that we were sisters and not mother and daughter. How did she do that?

My mother is a beauty expert who gave up her work when she turned 50, but even now she is a very active housewife.

She is a theta (a Japanese science of healing) healer. She started taking care of her skin much earlier, and it has become a part of her existence. She is a strong believer in all things natural, and has never coloured her hair or bleached her skin. She uses little or no make up, and has her own home remedies for everything. As a result, her body looks ten years younger and her skin at least 25 years younger than her real age!

According to my mother, it is very easy to make out the age of a woman: the more make-up she has on, the older she is. This summarizes why we apply make-up—to hide our flaws like puffy eyes, dark circles, scars and spots, uneven skin tone, dark lips, etc. Make-up also helps us to enhance our features like eyes, lips, cheekbones, etc. However, what you need to remember is that make-up is made up of chemicals and should not be overused. If you use too much make-up on a daily basis, your skin will start showing the ill effects very soon. These days, girls start wearing make-up very early on, even in their pre-teens. Parents must discourage this and allow it only for school functions, weddings, etc. Even then, kids should wear only basic, light make-up, as their fresh and beautiful skin does not need much make-up anyway!

Pre-teens

When you are in your pre-teens you should ideally not use any make-up unless you have to participate in some school function, go for weddings, etc.

Teens

Teens usually like to experiment with new things. This is the time when they go for body piercing, tattooing, hair colouring, etc. It is a crucial time of transition when you should experiment, but at the same time be careful not to damage your skin irrevocably. Avoid heavy make-up as much as you can, but if you like it then wear only kajal, and coloured lip gloss. And don't forget to take it off before sleeping.

Twenties

Jacqueline Fernandez is just 22 and is blessed with good skin. However, since she has begun acting and has had to apply heavy make-up, she has started taking care of her skin at this young age.

Jacqueline's beauty regime:
- Regular exercise and yoga
- Cleansing the skin everyday with Cetaphil
- Applying moisturizer with sunscreen
- Gently massaging the face for circulation
- Rubbing an ice cube over cleansed skin before moisturizing

Jacqueline is a slim and fit girl who wants to keep healthy in every possible way. Luckily, she has an extremely flexible body and enjoys what she does. She does yoga to look beautiful and feel energetic and fresh. Hence, the workouts that I have given her are very posture oriented and meditative. She works out whenever she is free and not caught up with work and tries to follow her routine at least three times a week. On the next page is the workout that I do with her. As you can see, Jacqueline does kriyas, Pranayam, and asanas which are good for both her body and appearance.

During your twenties, you need to make a conscious effort to take care of your skin, and follow your beauty regime. If

Jacqueline's exercise routine

Age: 22   Weight: 50 kilos   Sessions: 1 hour, three days a week
Target: To maintain weight and beauty.

Jacqueline follows the same routine three days a week.

1 A basic warm up for 5 to 6 minutes
2 Suryanamaskar: 20 to 30 rounds

Standing positions:

3 Vrikshasana: hold for 30 seconds on the right and left side, 2 sets
4 Tadasana: hold for 30 seconds on the right and left side, 2 sets
5 Trikonasana: hold for 30 seconds on the right and left side, 2 sets
6 Shishpadangustanasana: hold for 30 seconds on the right and left side, 2 sets
7 Garudasana: hold for 30 seconds on the right and left side, 1 set
8 Utkatasana: hold for 30 seconds

Sitting positions:

9 Ardha Matsyendrasana: hold for 30 seconds on the right and left side, 1 set
10 Paschimottanasana: hold for 30 seconds, 2 sets
11 Akarna Dhanurasana: hold for 30 seconds on the right and left side, 1 set
12 Ustrasana: hold for 30 seconds, 2 sets
13 Ugrasana: hold for 30 seconds, 2 sets
14 Supta Vajrasana: hold for 30 seconds, 1 set
15 Baddha Padmasana: hold for 30 seconds, 2 sets
16 Ardha Kapotasana: hold for 30 seconds on each leg

Supine positions:

17 Shavasana: 2 minutes
18 Sarvanganasana: hold for 30 second, 2 sets
19 Saral Matsyasana: hold for 20 seconds, 2 for sets
20 Poorna Halasana: hold for 30 second, 2 sets
21 Setubandhasana: hold for 30 seconds, 1 set

Prone positions:

22 Sarpasana: hold for 30 seconds, 1 set
23 Poorna Shalabhasana: hold for 30 seconds, 1 set
24 Naukasana on the stomach: hold for 30 seconds, 1 set
25 Dhanurasana: hold for 30 seconds, 1 set
26 Makarasana: 1 minute
27 Brahma Mudra: 3 rounds
28 Kapalbhati kriya: 50 strokes, 5 rounds
29 Bhastrika Pranayam: 3 to 5 rounds
30 Ujjayi Pranayam: 5 rounds
31 Anulom Vilom: 5 rounds
32 Bhramari: 5 rounds
33 Om chanting or any auspicious chant: 5 rounds
34 Shavasana: 2 minutes

you are alert and treat your skin well, you will reap the benefits later in your life. Use light make-up during the daytime like kajal and lip gloss, and heavy make-up only if necessary. You must take off all make-up before sleeping.

Dusky is in

It is no secret that Indians are obsessed with fair skin. The matrimonial ads are a testament to it, flooded as they are with searches for a 'milky white girl'. Fair skin is considered to be a trademark of beauty. But it is not necessarily so. The focus is fast changing from fair skin to a healthy glowing skin.

In India, there are four main types of skin colours: dark, medium also known as 'gehua' in Hindi, wheatish fair, and pinkish fair. Skin colour is genetic, and is what we inherit from our parents. The most important thing for me is to be comfortable in your skin. Be proud of what you have got, and make efforts to take care of it.

Look at the reigning actresses of Bollywood: Deepika, Bipasha, Priyanka, Sushmita, Rani, Kajol, none of whom are white in complexion. But aren't they popular? Are they not loved and admired by millions in India? Of course they are! And what about the models? Models, such as Madhu Sapre, Sheetal Malhar, Carol Gracias, Lakshmi Menon, are all dark skinned and have been consistently ruling the ramp. So there is no need to feel depressed or to go for skin-lightening treatments if you are not fair. The glow, that is a sign of healthy and happy skin, will do all the talking.

Thirties

Maria Goretti, the lovely former MTV veejay, is a hands-on mom of two children. Despite her busy schedule, Maria manages to look ravishing. She says, 'I start my day by drinking a big glass of mixed vegetable juice and then drink at least three big cups of green tea through the day. I love fruits and make it a point to eat one fruit a day if not more, and I make sure I never skip any of my meals. What keeps me fresh and going are catnaps and drinking plenty of water. And for that extra-healthy glow, I often eat chocolates!'

When you are in your thirties, your skin starts ageing visibly. Now you have no choice but to take care of your skin. Go for regular facials, at least once a month, and get it done only from a trained beautician. Use light make-up during the daytime, and heavy make-up only in the evenings or if necessary. As always, take it off before sleeping.

After Forty

If you did not take care of your skin while you were in your twenties or thirties, frankly there is not much you can do now. You have damaged your skin by now. But what you can still do

Sridevi's beauty mantra

- Drink a lot of water
- Do yoga regularly together with cardiovascular exercises
- Wash your face frequently
- Sleep well
- Think positive

is follow your beauty regime religiously, and avoid make-up at home. Your family already knows how you look! Use make-up only if you have to go out. Go for regular facials twice a month to help clean and tighten your skin.

Professional hazards

Unless you are in a profession that demands heavy make-up, you should try your best to avoid it. Film stars, models, airhostesses, TV journalists, and people in the service industry have no choice in this regard. They have to wear heavy make-up for their work, but this means that they also need to work harder on their skin. Your skin needs special care and nourishment. Try out these seven basic tricks to protect your skin, and keep it looking fresh and glowing:

1. If you have normal or dry skin, massage your skin with baby oil for 5 minutes in the morning after cleaning your face.
2. If you have oily skin, rub an ice cube on your face anytime during the day to open the pores clogged with make-up.
3. Splash your face with water whenever you can. It has a cleansing and cooling effect and also improves the circulation of blood in the face.
4. Always use good products suited for your skin type. Never use old cosmetics, and keep replacing them at least once in a year.
5. If you get dark circles, grate a raw potato together with its skin and apply the juice on your face. Wash it off after 10 minutes. Potato juice is a natural bleach and helps reduce dark circles as well.

6. Take 1 teaspoon of powdered rice and mix it with 1 teaspoon sugar crystals. Add a little water and apply it on your face whenever it feels dull. This acts as an excellent scrub for your skin and removes old and dead cells.
7. Repeat the beauty routine, depending upon your schedule and the level of exposure of your skin to the elements.

Tulip Joshi says, 'I have a four-pronged approach to skin care. I exercise regularly, sleep for at least 6 hours, take a nutritious diet, and maintain a healthy attitude towards everything around me. I have a simple beauty routine, but I follow this very diligently:

- I drink around 4 litres of water in a day.
- I use a face and body scrub once a week.
- Moisturize, moisturize, and moisturize. This is my skin care mantra. I moisturize my body from head to toe.
- For me, maintaining a high level of personal hygiene is also extremely important.

Taking care of your skin in changing seasons

Our skin reacts to the changes in the weather, and its needs are different in different weather conditions. Like in summer the skin naturally secretes oil, and you do not need to reapply the moisturizer. Similarly, in winter, the skin dries up much faster, and you need to regularly moisturize it. During rainy season, there is a lot of humidity in the air, and you need to keep your skin clean as well as dry. But what happens when the weather is changing? When it suddenly becomes very hot, your skin needs to adapt to the changed atmosphere outside, and might demand extra care during this period. You should learn to respond to your skin and follow the following rules:

- Summer to rainy: When the weather is changing from summer to rainy, you can treat your body with a refreshing massage. Rub your entire body with any

Body odour

Bad body odour can be a big turn off, especially during an interview, date, party, etc. Nobody likes someone who smells bad. In fact, sometimes it can be a huge source of embarrassment for the person with body odour.

What is body odour and why do some people have such unpleasant body odours? All of us sweat, and it is perfectly normal, natural, and healthy to do so. The most common areas which have sweat glands are the groin, scalp, and armpits. Through sweating, the body discards toxins out of the system. However, if we do not drink sufficient amounts of water, there is a greater concentration of salts in our perspiration, which produces a strong odour. Bad body odour can also be due to spicy food, stress, hot and humid weather, drinking hot beverages, wearing dirty nylon socks, etc. It can also be hereditary, or due to hormones, menopause, or illnesses.

What can you do? Drink at least 4 litres of water daily, and at regular intervals. Have regular baths, and dry yourself well after taking a shower. Use a cooling talcum powder before leaving the house. You should also change your footwear regularly and use cotton socks only instead of nylon ones, which do not let your feet breathe.

oil that suits you; like baby oil, olive oil, coconut oil, etc., for 10 minutes after taking a shower. Then rinse it, and pat your body dry.

- Rainy to winter: When there is a sudden chill in the air, we know that winter is around the corner. During this changing season, add 1 table spoon of honey in your bath water. It will make your skin smooth and soft.

- Winter to summer: As the new year progresses, summer creeps into most Indian cities. Summer is the longest season for most of us, and to welcome this harsh weather, make a pulp of any seasonal fruit like watermelon, papaya, etc., and apply it on your face. Leave it for 10 minutes, then wash it off.

Acne and pimples

Acne and pimples are an integral part of growing up just like hormones and puberty. It is a common problem faced by almost all teenagers and is mainly caused due to clogged pores, and may lead to pimples, or even scarring. Blackheads and whiteheads can also result in acne and pimples. If you want to remove blackheads at home, try this home remedy. Wet your face. Mix equal quantities of sugar and rawa (semolina) with water and rub it, upwards in clockwise motion on the affected area. Rub for 5 minutes and wash it off. Apply ice on your face to close the pores. Your dead cells will come out, and with them blackheads and whiteheads. Whiteheads can also form if you don't drink enough water as they arise from inside the skin.

My friend's teenaged daughter Rashmi refused to go to

a family dinner because she had an outbreak of pimples on her face. She was feeling too shy and embarrassed to face anyone. It is a big irritant for most teenagers, and can affect their self-esteem.

Acne are a result of your lifestyle, high level of hormone secretions during puberty, hormonal changes during periods, medications, too much oil in your food, reactions to medication or cosmetics, stress, bacterial infections, etc. People with oily skin are more prone to acne and pimples. They can also be caused by a recurrent upset stomach, having too much of oily, fried, or junk food.

Never touch a pimple or an acne. It will leave a mark

How we hate the big pimple staring back at us in the mirror on the eve of a party or a get together! And then we try to burst it open, hoping it will disappear or dry up faster. But this is the biggest mistake that you can do. You must never touch acne or a pimple. Just let it be, or even if you want to apply anything on it to dry it up, make sure you do not touch the pimple or press it in any way. If you touch it, it will surely leave a mark on your face. On the other hand, if you do not disturb it, it will go away in due course without scarring your skin. So if you want to avoid marks on your face, keep those itchy fingers away.

What can you do to control it?

There are many little things that you can do to keep acne and pimples at bay. Eat light and include a lot of fresh green vegetables and fluids in your diet. Have at least 4 litres of water every day. If you have oily skin and are prone to pimples, apply a neem-leaf pack throughout the year, and you will see a marked difference. People of all skin types can use seasonal fruit packs on their face for relief. If you already have a bad case of acne on your face, apply raw crushed garlic on top of it, and remove it after 5 minutes. This will help the acne to dry up faster.

My friend Hemali Punjabi is a 36-year-old HR manager. She has always been prone to pimples, and sometimes these would fill up her entire face. At such times, Hemali would avoid going out, as she felt embarrassed and unsure to face the world. However, Hemali's face totally cleared up when she started exercising and drinking more water. She has at least 4 to 5 litres of water every day, and no longer has any acne or pimples. By exercising and drinking water regularly, she managed to detox her body naturally, and throw out the toxins from her system. The effects are seen not only on her face but on her husband's face as well.☺

Bleaching and skin lightening

Many of us have a fascination for fair skin and try out different things like bleaching, skin lightening, etc. Bleach is a chemical which is used to lighten the skin tone. The common chemicals found in bleaches are ammonia, hydrogen peroxide, chlorine compounds, etc. Bleaching is becoming increasingly popular in India, even in small cities and towns. Excessive bleaching can be harmful for the skin. So do it if you want to, but limit it to only two or three times a year as it destroys the black pigment found in the top layer of the skin. The exposure of such skin to the harsh sunlight increases the probability of skin cancer. Pregnant women should never use bleach. However, you can bleach your skin naturally. And this does not damage your skin either. Potato juice is a natural bleaching agent. Grate a raw potato together with its skin and apply the juice on your face. Keep it on for 10 minutes, then wash it off. You can also use lime juice on your face regularly to lighten your skin tone.

What is skin lightening?

Some people want to go for intensive fairness procedures and opt for skin lightening. Skin lightening is a complicated process involving several stages of treatments. First the skin is peeled off. Thereafter, you are not allowed to be in the sun at all for the next 10 to 15 days till the new fairer skin comes out. It also involves applying packs, masks, and polishing the skin.

Skin lightening is a delicate and complex procedure, and should be performed only by experts. If you have to do it, make sure you go to a specialist and verify the credentials before you decide to take the plunge.

Exercises for skin

There are certain specific asanas in yoga which are extremely good for the skin. Deep breathing exercises and asanas enhance the flow of oxygen to the skin, help in balancing the hormones, and even keep your skin taut and toned. I recommend kriyas such as Jalneti and Sutraneti; asanas like Vipreetkarni, Sarvangasana, and Shirshasana; and Bhramari Pranayam for keeping your skin beautiful.

Hair care

Have you ever considered how important your hair is to your beauty? Ok, imagine how Sushmita Sen or Shilpa Shetty would look without their lovely mane? Yes, now you know what I mean. A good hairstyle can enhance your beauty just as a bad one can totally ruin the way you look. Hair is the outermost covering of most mammals, like humans, to protect them from the harsh conditions of the environment. It is an outgrowth from our skin and is made up of proteins called Keratin and amino acids.

Hair can be of different kinds, such as straight, wavy, or curly. In India, we mostly see straight or wavy hair, and it is again our genes which play an important role in the kind of hair that we have. Hair can also be categorized as normal, dry, and oily. Mostly people with oily skin have oily hair, dry skin have dry hair, and so on. Hair grows more in summers and also during the daytime.

How should I take care of my hair?

Just as you do with your skin, you need to take care of your hair regularly. Avoid hot water for washing hair, even in winter, as it damages your cuticles. Once I met a girl whose shoulder was full of pimples. On inquiring I found out that she loved to shower in hot water. As a result, she had scalded her back and even developed pimples due to the excessive heat on the skin. So remember to use only lukewarm water for washing your hair.

Use an organic or natural shampoo suited for your skin type, and don't forget to apply conditioner every time you wash your hair. The conditioner should never penetrate your scalp. Ensure that you apply it only on the ends and not on the roots of your hair. Leave it for 5 minutes then wash away completely with at least a bucket full of water.

There are many misconceptions about oil massages. Some say it is good while others claim that there is no need for oil massages. I recommend warm-oil massages at least twice a week. Let me explain why it is good for your hair. When you massage your scalp with oil, the blood circulation increases and it gets more oxygen. This makes your hair soft, and also helps you to relax. However, the correct way to massage your hair is in alternate, clockwise, and anti-clockwise directions using your finger tips. If you do not like oiling your hair, you can avoid it during summers as the scalp secretes more natural oils during this season. Instead, you can use the homemade natural pack, which I use myself and recommend for all hair types. This is extremely good for your hair and can be used in all seasons to get the hair you dream of.

Mix the paste of 1 bunch of fresh methi leaves (tonic), 1 crushed beetroot (colour), 6 to 8 crushed shoe flowers (softness), 4 tablespoons of multani mitti (cleaning), 1 full egg (protein; you can leave this if you cannot stand the smell), and apply it on your hair. Keep this pack on for 20 to 25 minutes only and not longer. Wash it off with lukewarm water. If you do not like oiling your hair, add one tablespoon of oil to this pack before applying. I feel this pack is excellent for hair growth and also lends a natural rich sheen to your hair.

Why does hair fall?

Have you ever woken up to find a cluster of hair on your pillows? Or have you ever combed your hair and found a bunch of strands sticking to the comb? There cannot be a worse beginning to the day. Hair fall can be really depressing. It makes your hair look thin and lifeless. So why does hair fall? There are many reasons for hair fall, like lack of vitamin C in your body, change of climate, hormonal imbalances, chronic diseases, heat and humidity, dirt, unsuitable hair products, stress, unhealthy diet, lack of sleep, pregnancy, etc. Sudden hair fall leading to baldness, is hereditary and especially common in men. It can also be caused, or aggravated, by the excessive use of hairsprays, gels, hair colours, etc. Most of these men had a healthy crop during their youth but with progressing age, they are faced with consistent hair fall and a receding hairline.

Hair fall of around forty strands a day is considered to be normal. But more than that is a cause of worry and should be dealt with urgently. In India, it is usually seen that hair falls more between June to September, and less in winters. Dandruff can also cause hair fall especially in the cold, winter months. Wash your hair only twice a week in winters as it can rob your hair of the little natural oil secreted.

What can you do to control hair fall? My mother recommends four basic measures to control hair fall. First, you need to make sure that you are having a regular and a balanced diet which includes dal, green vegetables, fish, eggs, aloe vera, etc. You can supplement your diet by including vitamin C and vitamin E. Take the vitamins every morning after breakfast for forty days at a stretch. Then take a break of ten days and continue again. Second, brush your hair from the front as well as the back in the morning and before going to bed, with a vent brush. This will improve the circulation of blood to the scalp. Third, sleep well and exercise regularly. This helps to open up the pores and remove toxins through sweat. Last, follow your routine of cleaning and oiling (or applying the hair pack) regularly. Do this for two to three months and you will have happier mornings.

Mundan in India

A mundan is a popular and an important ceremony among Hindus in India. It is the first haircut of the baby usually done in either the first year or the third year. A priest is called to conduct the rituals according to the traditions and a barber is called to shave off the hair, sometimes leaving a clump of hair at the back of the head. Some of this hair is offered to the sacred rivers in holy cities like Haridwar and Varanasi. A paste of turmeric and sandalwood is, sometimes, applied on the head after the mundan, to cool down the head and to cure nicks and cuts. It is believed that the unwanted traits from your past lives can be removed through this ritual. Mundan also promotes the circulation of blood to the head, and hence promotes hair growth. No wonder the hair that comes out after mundan is usually thicker and healthier.

Hair colouring

It is fun to experiment with different kinds of looks, and that includes different hair colours as well. You must have seen college going kids or even older people with purple, orange, or pink hair. Bebo too has pink hair for a song in *Tashan*. There are many ways to colour your hair. You can go the natural way and use henna or the hair pack I suggested for a nice sheen to your mane. Regular use of henna or the hair pack can bring about a natural burgundy colour.

If you want to go for other hair colouring products, go for a good product, and don't forget to do a skin test before applying it all over your head. Make sure that your hair colour is ammonia free, or contains as little chemicals as possible. Also, make sure that the hair colour never touches your scalp. However, since all these products contain strong chemicals, pregnant women must never colour, perm, or streak their hair.

Exercises for hair

Just as with the skin, there are some exercises that I especially recommend for the hair. Asanas such as Sarvangasana, Poorna Halasana, Shirshasana, and Matsyasana improve the circulation of blood to the head and boost hair growth. You can also do kriyas like Kapalbhati, Jalneti, and Sutraneti and breathing exercises, such as Anulom Vilom Pranayam and Bhramari Pranayam to have thick, healthy hair.

Eye care

Eyes are said to be the most delicate and precious parts of our body. You must clean your eyes every time you wash your face, and remove all make-up before sleeping. Also, drink a lot of water, use sunglasses whenever you go out, and cut down on alcohol or caffeine. If you do not take care of your body, it will show as dark circles around your eyes. Interestingly, the signs of ageing are first visible around the eyes. It might start with some fine lines around the eyes, followed by crow's feet, dark circles, puffiness under the eyes, etc.

If you want to avoid crow's feet, never rub your eyes

vigorously. Remember, the skin around your eyes is delicate and once it gets damaged, it can never be repaired. The broken tissues remain broken and do not get replaced. Use a good eye drop once a week to lubricate your eyes.

Dark circles and puffy eyes are a result of small and broken tissues around your eyes. This can be caused due to fluid retention, allergies, wrong medication, hereditary reasons, lack of sleep, stress, ageing, pregnancy, improper diet, bad make-up, etc. At night before sleeping, apply an under-eye cream, but be careful not to leave it on for more than 2 minutes. Then dab it off with a wet cotton pad. Never sleep with the under-eye cream on, or rub it inside the skin around your eye. If you have an itching sensation in your eyes, and you have to rub your eyes, use the insides of your palm instead of your fingers. You can also try these home remedies to cure puffiness and dark circles:

- Soak 7 sultanas overnight and drink it with water in the morning.
- Apply an ice or cucumber pack on your eyes for 10 minutes.
- You can also try raw potato juice or moist tea bags, all stored and kept ready in the refrigerator. Apply it when you are tired or come back home after a long day.
- One of the interesting ways that I used to deal with dark circles is lying down with the head free falling from the bed for 5 to 10 minutes after waking up. This enhances the blood circulation to the head and the eyes, and helps reduce dark circles around the eyes.

If you have dry eyes due to working on the computer for long without breaks, refrain from using or getting too close

Contact lenses

Many of us use contact lenses instead of glasses and even use coloured lenses. Since eyes are the most delicate part of our body, we need to take extra care to keep them healthy. And if you use contact lenses daily then you need to be extra conscious. You might ask as to why lenses need special care and not glasses. This is because lenses stick to our eyes and are in direct contact with them all the time. So if you do not clean your lenses properly, and there is some dirt on the surface, it will immediately affect your eyes. On the other hand, glasses are at a distance and not in direct contact with the eyes. Glasses also allow the eyes to breathe, and in fact shield them from dust and pollution. So make sure that you clean your lenses after every 4 hours, and replace them as and when required.

to hair dryers, heaters, blowers, etc., as they will further dry up your eyes. Instead, use a good eye drop or any of the eye packs that I have recommended.

Exercises for eyes

Kriyas like Tratak and eye rotations are extremely beneficial for the eyes. I also recommend asanas, such as Vipreetkarni, Sarvangasana, Matsyasana, and Brahma Mudra, which work on your eye muscles. My eyes feel relaxed and fresh after I do these asanas. These are extremely good for people whose work involves straining their eyes like photographers, doctors, engineers, bankers, pilots, etc. In fact, these exercises are useful for anyone working on the computer for long and can help relax the eye muscles after a long day.

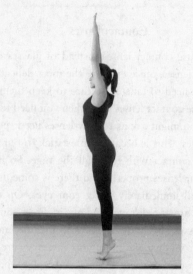

Tadasana

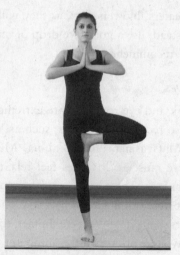

Vrikshasana

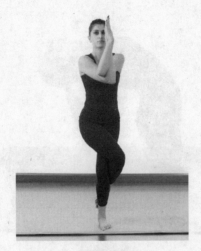

Garudasana

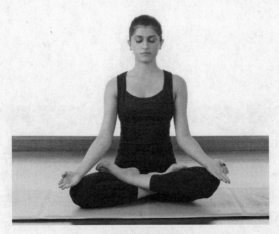

Padmasana

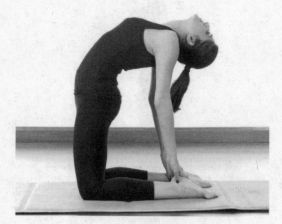

Ustrasana

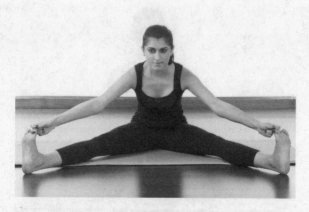

Ugrasana

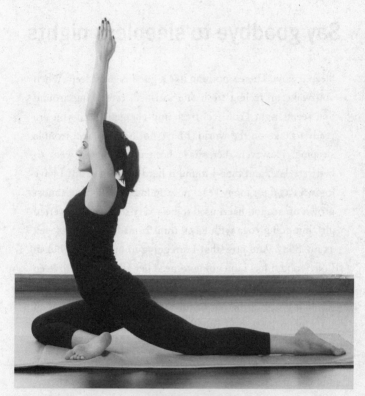

Ardha Kapotasana

7

Say goodbye to sleepless nights

Sleep…wow. There's nothing like a good night's sleep. When you wake up feeling fresh and satisfied, everything around you seems right. You feel fresh and energetic, and you are ready to take on the world. I have not had any real trouble sleeping. However, there have been days when I went to bed very late, and then I found it hard to sleep easily. I have known Payal for many years now. In fact, I feel I have almost grown up around her. I used to be a very shy and introverted girl, but doing yoga with Payal transformed my mind as well as my body. And now that I am going to make my debut in Bollywood, I feel I am going to need her all the more to keep fit and beautiful despite the hectic schedules and late nights. To help me sleep better, Payal made me do 500 strokes of Kapalbhati kriya in 4 rounds. This really helped to cleanse my body. So I guess even if you have hectic schedules, you can take the help of certain exercises and wake up feeling fresh and energized.

Zoa Morani

Sleep for me, and I'm sure for many of you, is one of the most important factors that make a great day. Who wants to wake up groggy and exhausted and that too right in the morning? Sleep is just as important as exercise for the body. Our mind and body need to rest to be rejuvenated, and to prepare for the challenges that the next day throws at us. There are a few people I know who can manage with less sleep. They have trained their bodies accordingly and can do with 3 to 5 hours of sleep. However, most of us crave for a good 6 to 8 hours of sleep. Personally, if I do not get my 8 hours of sleep, I feel very cranky and tired. On top of it, I don't feel enthusiastic about doing anything. Some of you might find it hard to concentrate or focus on what you are doing, feel irritable, snappy, and end up picking fights. If this pattern of irregular or disturbed sleep continues, it can eventually change your appearance. You might end up having dark circles under your eyes, and it can even lead to hair loss. So there are physical ramifications of lack of sleep as well.

Getting to your 'ultimate sleep'

Once my client Ambika Roye said to me: 'Wow! I got the best sleep today. This is how I want to wake up every day. All of us yearn to wake up with a smile and feeling as fresh as a flower. A good night's sleep is when you wake up not feeling tired but refreshed. And isn't this the very purpose of sleeping? To give the mind and body rest?

My 'ultimate sleep' as I call it is dreamless and undisturbed, when you sleep at a stretch and don't remember anything of what happened during the night. You sleep and get up without realizing the time, thinking it was just moments before when you got into bed. The reason for this lies in the very fundamentals of sleeping. What happens when we sleep? Every time you go to sleep, your organs slow down, your thought processes cease or more appropriately your conscious mind stops working, your breathing becomes regular and calm, and so on. Now if you keep on waking up in between during the night, you are likely to disturb this sleeping pattern. Every time you get up during the night and try to sleep again, the body has to go through the entire process again. As a result, the net effective sleep that you get is much less than what you would have got if you had slept at a stretch.

Once a friend asked me: 'Payal, how do I know whether I am getting my ultimate sleep? What are the signs?' The answer lies in your behaviour. If you are not cranky, irritable, drowsy, angry, etc., right in the morning, I would say you have got your ultimate sleep. It's really simple actually. If you do not give the body its due, it reacts to show that it's not happy. And it can express its displeasure in more ways than one. So if you are snapping at your children or your maid in the morning, feeling like you've just ended your day rather than beginning it, are not in the mood for jokes or a little harmless teasing, you have not got your due sleep. Here I would like to add that some people take a little longer to get up, may be half an hour or so, before they feel active or fresh. This is perfectly normal, and not a sign of sleep debt.

How much sleep is good sleep?

Too much of one thing is never good. Just as it is important to exercise to be active, it is equally essential to get a good night's sleep to allow the mind and the body to relax. After a normal day which is hectic for most of us nowadays, the body needs to rest and recuperate to prepare for the next day.

I always tell my clients that sleep is a reflection of how your day has gone by, both in terms of the quantity and the quality. If you wake up feeling tired, irritable, or angry chances are that you have not given your body its deserved time off. Under normal circumstances, 6 to 8 hours should do the trick. But this is not enough in all cases. Infants, toddlers, school kids, etc., need many more hours of sleep to allow the healthy development of the brain and the body. Similarly, when you are unwell you need to sleep more to help your body fight back. Sleep helps to strengthen the immune system, which is under attack whenever you have some infection or disorder. In fact, if you are getting your required sleep, you are less likely than others to fall prey to germs or diseases. Interestingly, most animals simply sleep off their illness. Such is the power of a good restful sleep.

My sleep table

Age	General Lifestyle	Required Hours of Sleep	Nap's During a Day
0–6 months	easy	all day; up only when hungry	All day
6–12 months	starts getting a little active, cries at intervals	16–17 hrs a day	Could be any time
1–2 years	baby feels tired as she/ he has started walking and understanding the surroundings	16–17 hrs	Could be any time
3–5 years	started going to play school, life has changed	16–17 hrs	Could be any time

Age	General Lifestyle	Required Hours of Sleep	Nap's During a Day
5–9 years	has started to read and write hours of school are now fixed	Night– 10 hours	1–2
9–12 years	hectic school life; full of energy	Night– 10 hours	1–2 if required
13–19 years	very busy in studies and extracurricular activities	Night–8 to 10 hours	1–2
20's	busy and looking out for fun	8 hours	1–2
30's	busy yet more responsible	8 hours	2–3
40's	busy and responsibilities increases further	7–8 hours	2–3
50's	life eases	7–8 hours	2–3

As you grow older, your sleep becomes lighter. Most people in their fifties and sixties cannot get restful sleep, or sleep at a stretch no matter how much they try. I remember my mother craving for the 'teenager's sleep' as she called it, when you can just doze off before you can count up to ten. So if you are trying to sneak into the house quietly after a late night, you are more likely to be caught by your grandparents than your parents!

Sleeping too much is not recommended as it makes you dull, lazy, and sluggish. If you oversleep, your body movements slow down, and the brain is not as alert as it should be. On the other hand, if you don't get your required hours of sleep, you feel tired, drowsy, cranky, and inattentive, and cannot concentrate. This is the reason why I strongly recommend my clients to sleep well before they have to take an exam, go for an interview, take a screen test, or even when they have to drive. So many accidents on the roads are due to the fact that the drivers were not able to react well in time. They had not slept well and were simply feeling drowsy at the wheels, putting precious lives at risk.

Rameet Gidwani, a 28-year-old, is an Assistant General Manager a leading Mumbai hotel. Given her job profile, she has to stand almost 10 hours a day, mostly from 9 am to 7 pm. Her job is very strenuous, being both mental and physical in nature. So by the time Meet gets home, she feels very tired, and has difficulty getting good sleep on most nights. She can barely get 2 to 3 hours at a stretch, and keeps on waking up throughout the night. She was tired, irritable, and frustrated.

Almost six months back, Meet came to me and started doing yoga. I made her do Bhramari Pranayam, Shavasana, Parvatasana, and Suryanamaskars. These exercises improved the blood circulation in her body, and helped her to relax. Suryanamaskars enhance the cardio vascular endurance as well as the flexibility of the muscles. She has since experienced a change in her sleep pattern, and can now sleep 6 to 7 hours at a stretch. As a result, Meet feels energetic and happy in the mornings. This has made a lot of difference in her life, and has helped her perform better at work.

So this is what sleep does: it keeps you healthy, beautiful

and sharp. It is as important as eating and exercising. And the way you sleep, and how much, is just as relevant to bring about the best results.

I sleep 7 hours at a stretch and still feel tired!

Well, it also matters where you sleep. It is important to make sure that the place where you spend 6 to 8 hours in a day is ideal for you. A lot of people like to sleep in water beds or soft mattresses, which are really bad for the body especially the back. The truth is, the harder the surface, the better it is. If you want to get your ultimate sleep, make sure that your mattress is firm and not too soft. Also, remember to discard your old mattresses after 4 to 5 years.

A lot of people have trouble going off to sleep at night even though they are perfectly normal and do not suffer from any sleeping disorders. In most such cases, I have seen that these people lead a sedentary life with very little physical activity. Siddhartha Mehta, 19, is a fresher in college and is completely addicted to the internet. He loves to chat with

Tips to get your ultimate sleep

- Listen to some soothing music
- Take a lukewarm bath before going to bed
- Keep your bedroom, or where you sleep clean
- Remove the clutter around your bed
- Use aroma candles with lavender or any other fragrant oil that you like
- Wash your feet before sleeping

his friends, play online games on the computer, and doesn't realize how the hours pass by. As a result, most of the time he's holed up in his bedroom and doesn't like to meet people or venture outdoors. Things came to a head when he wanted to have his meals in his room too. He became lazy and a sluggish couch potato. Doing anything became an effort for him. He didn't want to leave his room, was unsocial, didn't talk much, invited friends to his room instead of going out with them, argued and didn't listen to his parents. He also had problems sleeping as he was lazy, with no physical activity.

The solution to such users is simple: you need to work to sleep. Here I do not mean that you need to get a job, but simply that you need to exert your body to sleep well in the night. When the body is resting the entire day, with little to do, your muscles do not feel tired and hence there is no real need to sleep and get refreshed. So start with any one activity: take up a sport, go for an hour of brisk walk, or if you have to be at home then doing something as basic as cooking, dusting, cleaning your wardrobe, can also help you sleep better in the night.

What not to do for a good night's sleep

- Eat heavy or greasy food at night
- Eat fermented food like idli, dosa, maida, etc.
- No cold fruits like watermelon, pineapple, musk melon, etc.
- Never watch horror movies in the night or unpleasant shows on TV with violence, blood, or gore

You cannot sleep when you have the time and feel sleepy when you can't

Aanchal Patel is a 33-year-old magazine journalist. Every month during the magazine closing time, the work gets hectic and days easily melt away into nights without Aanchal realizing it. As a result, when she wakes up after the little sleep that she gets, she feels drained and finds it difficult to concentrate on her work. What is worse is that sometimes she is so tired that she just cannot sleep and this really irritates her as she feels that the precious few hours are slipping away and she cannot do anything about it.

Many people I have met feel that they cannot sleep well when they want to, like on the weekends or holidays, but feel extremely sleepy during crunch times like during tough deadlines etc., when they would like to be active. A lot of students experience this phenomenon—they can't keep their eyes open while studying for their exams but when the examination is over, they cannot sleep no matter how much they try even though they are sleep deprived. There are two main reasons for this. First, your body has to get acclimatized to the new sleep pattern, which in this case means sleeping for lesser number of hours. And so it'll takes some time to get back to normal routine. Second, now you do not feel as tired or stressed as before, so your mind does not need as much rest as it does during a taxing time or a crisis. Remember, you need to work to sleep? So what do you do? Play or do some physical activity and get your body tired. You will not only feel refreshed, but will also be able to sleep better.

Tips for students to sleep well during exams

- Have a glass of milk with honey at night
- Don't have too much tea or coffee at night
- Concentrate on studying instead of thinking too much about the exam
- Make a pattern—either study late in the night or early in the morning—depending on whether you are a night person or a morning person; but don't do both
- When you are very stressed, calm down and talk to yourself
- You need to take a break. Do whatever you like for 30 minutes in between to relax: like listening to music, playing videogames, playing sports.

Sleep disorders

Everybody has a rough day, when things go wrong, or not as you would have liked or planned. Like when you have a cold, blocked nose, and are coughing or sneezing all night long. Or you are stressed about some problem at home or at work, and have trouble sleeping. On such days you can try one of the tips to sleep well, and you will experience the results. This is perfectly normal, and does not mean that you have a sleeping disorder. But when you face problems in sleeping on a regular basis, you might have a sleeping disorder. I have a simple test for this: I ask my clients when they last slept really well or got the 'ultimate sleep' as I call it. If the answer is: 'I can't remember when was the last time' or 'Let me think...not in a long time' is when you might have a sleeping problem.

My husband snores so loudly! I'm thinking of leaving him.

Why do people snore? Snoring is caused by a blockage in your nasal airway, either from poor sleep posture, excess weight or physical abnormalities of your throat. A narrow airway gets in the way of smooth breathing and creates the sound of snoring.

There are many self-help remedies and cures for snoring. Snoring is more common in men than in women as men have narrower air passages. If you snore mildly, sleeping on your side, elevating the head of your bed, or losing weight may stop the snoring. Or it could be cold, sinuses, asthma, infection, or wrong sleep posture that makes you snore. Hereditary reasons and heavy medication can make you snore; so avoid alcohol at night. You can do Jalneti, Vaman kriya, and Bhramari Pranayam to open your nasal and throat cavities.

Snoring can affect your relationships in a big way. In the West there are divorces due to snoring. Even in India, it can cause strained relationships between couples. When your partner is not able to sleep well on a regular basis it causes irritability and you can end up fighting over small issues. Don't give up trying to find a solution for your snoring—it will make you and your partner sleep better. And of course, the days too would be merrier!

What is insomnia?

When you cannot sleep well for more than a few odd days, it is referred to as insomnia. Any of us can have short-term insomnia—like during weddings, examinations, project submissions, illnesses—when we cannot sleep well for a few days. This is also known as acute insomnia. However, if you cannot sleep for at least three nights per week for more than a month at a stretch, it is called chronic insomnia. Chronic insomnia can adversely affect your work, relationships, and health, and needs to be treated as soon as possible.

Rina Shah is a 16-year-old young and vivacious girl. She could not sleep well for around two weeks when her elder sister was getting married. There were cousins and guests in the house, and most nights they would end up chatting till late. They had planned a rocking ladies night with song and dance performances by everybody, and would practise for it for hours. But after the wedding was over and when all the guests had left, it was back to normal. Still, Rina could not sleep normally at least for a few days.

Insomnia often is the harbinger of other serious problems in your lives. Your insomnia might be a symptom of a more significant sleep problem. It might be a precursor for dealing with physical, mental, or emotional challenges. In some cases, your inability to fall asleep or stay asleep in the night might be related to your partner's snoring, an urgent situation at work, or a difficult family issue. Whatever the cause of your insomnia might be, you can get it cured to sleep better and feel better.

Oh no! Not in the night please!

Most of us today sleep with one person but more than one gadgets. No seriously...don't you sleep with your mobile phone next to your pillow or your ear, and your laptop on the bedside? How often do we not talk over the phone in our beds? It's lovely and 'oh so mushy' to talk to your lover lying on your pillow but you might change your mind when you learn of the side effects. Heavy radiations coming out of mobile phones, laptops, and gadgets affect the weaker parts of the body like the eyesight, heart, brain, and even your sexual organs! It is also really harmful for pregnant women. Not only do electronic gadgets hamper your sleep, but they can also cause serious damage to your health in the long run.

What happens when the phone rings in the middle of the night? Obviously, you get up to answer the phone and your sleep is disturbed. The mind and body that were resting by shutting off from the outside world are rudely awakened, and forced to connect with the outside world again. As a result, the next morning when you wake up, you feel tired and irritated. I strongly recommend that you keep electronics out of your bedroom. Try it for a week and you will feel the difference.

A new mommy? Here's what you should do

- Remember that you have entered a new phase in your life; you might want to run back to your normal sleep pattern post delivery, but it is not possible for at least one year.
- Learn to take quick naps when your baby's sleeping. This is something that you have to train yourself to do. Such power naps will keep you active and fresh during these difficult months.
- Don't run to do errands when your baby is asleep; this is your sleeping time too!
- Train the baby to follow a consistent sleep pattern, so that you can adjust to it yourself.

Get back home a flower not a thorn

Actor Tulip Joshi is in her thirties and totally chilled out. Although she is in a very competitive profession, she manages to stay relaxed as her friends and family help her stay grounded. Tulip is content with what she has and enjoys her work. She does roles that she likes without blindly following the trend and signing movies one after the other. No wonder she is contented and a happy-go-lucky person.

Problems, deadlines, and worries are a part of all our lives. The bare truth of our lives today is that all of us have a minimum baggage that we need to carry on a daily basis. And this does not only apply to working people. There is a very popular misconception that housewives have less number of things to worry about. However, the fact of the matter is that most housewives who have to run the house are on their toes from morning till night, making sure the maids work properly, the kids are sent off to school, the husband gets what he needs and is off to work, everybody is fed on time, getting the groceries, etc.

What I want to say here is that do not pile on more than required on your plate. Always be positive in life, and leave the negativities out of the house. In the course of your day, you might meet some people you don't like, you might hear some gossip, might experience work-related stress, etc. You already have enough things to worry about so don't poke your nose in things that you can do without, and don't bring home extra worries. This will not only help you to be calm and peaceful, and enjoy your time with your family, but also ensure that you get a restful sleep at night. The quality of sleep that we get, is linked with what we do and think, so the more that you filter your thoughts and accept only positives, the better you will be able to sleep at night. Bring home happiness, not extra worries.

A basic routine for getting your ultimate sleep

Basic precautions:

1. Never workout on a heavy stomach.
2. Exercise preferably 2 hours after your breakfast and 4 hours after your lunch.
3. Drink at least 4 to 5 litres of water in a day to avoid constipation and indigestion.
4. There should be a break of at least 10 seconds between each asana in the sequence.
5. If you have any kind of ailments or health related issues please consult your doctor before doing any exercise or do it under the guidance of a yoga teacher.

Where: Choose a place which has fresh air circulation preferably a garden, a terrace, or a workout place in your house. For Jalneti, you need a wash basin.

What you need: A yoga mat, and a hand, or a face towel. For Jalneti, you need the pot.

Duration: 30 minutes

1. Jalneti kriya: twice a week, only during the morning on an empty stomach
2. Vipreetkarni: hold for 20 seconds, 3 sets, six days a week
3. Sarvangasana: hold for 20 seconds, 3 sets, six days a week
4. Parvatasana: hold for 20 seconds, 3 sets, six days a week
5. Chandrabedhan: 3 rounds

6. Bhramari: 10 rounds
7. Om chanting: 10 rounds
8. Shavasana: 10 minutes

How to sleep well after late-night parties: How to cope with sleep deficit

- Partying is good for fun but not to run away from reality. I would say you should not party more than 3 times a week. You sleep late, eat out late. To make up for your sleep debt, take a quick nap in the afternoon.
- Drink to sleep: Really stressed, and so tired that you can't sleep? Have one glass of wine or one glass of beer, not more, and it will help you sleep well. This tip works only when you are really exhausted, and you are a social drinker.

Are you stressed?

Stress is one of the most commonly used terms today, in city life. If you have a lot of work pressure you are stressed, if there are many guests in your home you get stressed, if it is festival time or hectic celebrations then again we feel stressed. We have to juggle different roles at home and at work, and sometimes it gets too much to handle. In order to stay on top of things, you need to be mentally and physically fit. When you are stressed your sleep also gets disturbed. Although sleep is one of the best ways to relieve stress, it is something that often gets compromised under stress. In the previous pages we talked about how yoga is good for sleep. Yoga is also beneficial for stress as it helps attain mental and physical balance. It not only keeps you physically fit but can help you to keep your mind calm and alert.

What is stress?

Stress is the combination of physical and mental overload that disturbs the normal functioning of the body. There are times when you just feel like you have had enough and cannot go on anymore. This state is known as stress. Interestingly, many people feel that they can perform better under stress. This may be so as the stress hormones like cortisol, growth hormone (GH), etc., give a boost to the coping mechanism. When you cannot handle things properly due to a new scenario, unorganized or unplanned work, a weak nervous system, sudden pressure at work or at home, competition, etc., you can feel stressed. Students usually feel stressed out during examinations, while working professionals feel the heat mostly during projects or deadlines. The point is that everybody experiences it sometime or the other but it becomes a problem if it starts occurring frequently or without any break. In that case, it starts affecting your sleep and can hamper your health, causing diseases.

Stressed? Me? No way! I know it sounds strange. But being a wife, a mother, and a politician I cannot afford to let stress become a part of my life. I like to be positive and go with the flow. I live in the present and take on each day as it comes.

I still remember the day, a year back when I simply cycled my way to Payal's studio Cosmic Fusion. I am like that. I love outdoor physical activities, especially cycling. Of course, since I am an MP, I have to be careful, but cycling is a great stress buster for me and I do it whenever I can. It is an environmental friendly way to travel and I feel there is really no age to pick up your good old bike. Besides, Payal's place was near my house. That was the first time I met Payal. And the moment I entered her studio, I felt really refreshed. So the second important thing for me to be stress free is to have a clean, soothing environment around me. This is what I try to incorporate at home as well. It really works wonders for me. The studio was done up beautifully, and it instantly had a calming effect on me. And of course I exercise regularly to let the stress out of my mind and my body. These simple choices I made in my life have helped me significantly. You could also try out my tips and lead a happy, stress free life.

Priya Dutt **Priya Dutt**

What are the signs of stress?

Mita Sharma is a successful 38-year-old lawyer. Being in a demanding profession, Mita learnt the ropes quickly, and started being respected for her work. Soon she started a law firm with her friend and things were progressing smoothly. However, two months back her friend left the company due to some personal reason and since then Mita has had to manage everything on her own. Earlier she worked till 10 pm now she cannot finish even by 1 am. She hasn't been able to find a replacement and now clear signs of stress have started showing. Mita has regular headaches and sleeps very little. She has also had instances of palpitation lately. Clearly, Mita's body is trying to tell her that it needs a break.

There are many signs of stress like sweating in the palms and the feet, high blood pressure, feeling exhausted all the time, having regular headaches or acidity, body tremors, insomnia, feeling thirsty all the time, allergies, sudden hair fall or greying, memory loss, infertility, etc. In times of stress, the lactic acid secretion in the muscles, especially around your neck and shoulders increases, making you feel tired and drained. Your heart starts beating faster, and this can result in palpitation or hypertension. Everybody has a rough patch now and then, but if things don't improve at all, your body can display signs of stress.

I will now share with you my five principles of dealing with stress and enjoying peaceful sleep in the night.

Principle one: Accept it. Shouting is not a solution

Ayesha Kapoor is a 25-year-old newly married woman in Delhi. Since she got married in early 2010, she has not been getting along well with her mother-in-law, who she feels is too interfering. Ayesha works in a public relations firm and when she gets back home, she feels exhausted and feels like relaxing, but unfortunately since the two don't get along, they keep arguing on and off. As a result, Ayesha has been feeling very stressed out lately.

The first step towards dealing with stress is accepting the situation and then finding a solution. If you want an easy going happy life, you need to accept the challenges that come your way and then find a way around them. A positive attitude of looking at things certainly goes a long way in dealing with most of the problems in our lives. So throw out the negativities like greed, anger, fear, jealousy, competition, inferiority complexes, low self-esteem, discrimination, ego, anxiety, etc. and your life will become much simpler and happier.

Another thing that you can train yourself to do is play roles. Women should learn to seamlessly and effortlessly fit into the roles of girlfriend, wife, mother, etc., while men can fit into the roles of boyfriends, husbands, and fathers. In today's world, you have to learn to switch off and switch on according to the situation.

Principle two: Plan how to go about it and work towards it

When Rajiv Sethi, a 29-year-old entrepreneur had sudden losses in his business, he just didn't know how to handle the situation. Initially, he didn't know who to turn to or what to do. But he kept on trying new ideas, and after a fortnight when he found a solution to deal with the situation, he felt less stressed out.

It is extremely important to be level headed and calm in order to handle any kind of a crisis situation. Only then can you plan a way out of the mess and follow it too. On the other hand, if you live life in an organized manner, chances are you will be able to avoid most stressful situations. Like when you know your deadline is a week away, don't wait till the last day to finish your work. Plan in advance and work towards it regularly to avoid stress and sleepless nights during the crunch time.

Principle three: Remember that it is only a temporary phase

A lot of situations like examinations, sudden advent of house guests, weddings in the family, etc., are a temporary phase in your life and you should always remind yourself of that.

Pooja Thapar is an 18-year-old college-going girl. During her annual examination she used to feel very exhausted and would have sleepless nights worrying about her scores. But when her friend reminded her about the holiday trip she was planning after the examinations, she felt encouraged. She started working hard focusing on the merry times to come after the examinations and this actually helped her score better. The thought of a break from studying for long hours relieved her somewhat of the constant mental pressure.

Principle four: Use your experience to be better prepared

When Nina Subramaniam had her first child in America at 24, she was alone with her husband, without any family or help. She had never imagined that motherhood was such hard work, so when the new baby arrived she felt exhausted and irritated most of the time, as she barely got any sleep. Her husband took two weeks off from work to help her, but after that she was on her own and struggling to cope. However, when Nina had her second child, she had planned everything in advance right from the food to the laundry, to baby care, and this time round it seemed like a cakewalk. She had trained herself to take power naps as she called them, and felt fresh most of the time. This was because Nina had put her experience to good use to avoid stress. You too can learn from your own, or even better others' experiences to handle tough situations better.

Principle five: Learn to say no. Don't commit to more than you can deliver

It is very important to learn to say *no* if you know you cannot do something. Don't be too shy or over-confident to say yes and then torture yourself later. Many people have this habit of saying yes to everything, but when it comes to delivering on the promise, they struggle and consequently get stressed. Remember that one person can't do everything and that you need to delegate work. My friend Rhea Chandra is a 24-year-old engineer working with an MNC. Her problem is that she cannot say no to her boss for anything. As a result, she ends up doing, not only her work, but most of her boss' as well. Things got so bad that last week she passed out due to heat and exhaustion. Let's face it. Superman and superwoman exist only in books and films. There's no point inviting stress into our lives.

Stress and depression

It is generally believed that stress and depression are inter-related. Depression is mostly the fallout of a stressful situation. You must have all heard about the recent incident of Viveka Babaji's death, which surprised her friends and family alike.

The common reasons for depression are death of a loved one, loss of name, fame, money, break up of a relationship, a traumatic experience, etc. I am not saying that this is always the case. Sometimes, you can be depressed without any concrete reason. However, the fact remains that severe stressful relations can end up in depression. This is all the more reason to find solutions for stress and to learn to handle trying situations.

Yoga for acute stress

If you feel stressed out regularly, you can follow this simple workout to relieve stress. It not only helps to make you feel relaxed but also helps you sleep better. You need to follow the routine six days in a week. Continue doing it till you feel relieved. In fact, you can continue doing it, as it will keep you relaxed, calm, alert, and improve your mental and physical balance.

1. Kapalbhati: 50 to 120 strokes, 3 rounds
2. Shavasana: 10 minutes
3. Sukhasana: 2–5 minutes
4. Bhramari Pranayam: 12 rounds
5. Anulom Vilom Pranayam: 12 rounds
6. Om chanting or any other auspicious chant: 12 times

Ways to relax the mind and the body

Some things you can try to relax yourself are:

- going to a spa
- any kind of exercise
- running
- cooking
- playing with pets
- watching movies
- listening to music
- dancing
- washing clothes
- long walks
- long drives
- trekking
- cleaning
- gardening, farming
- painting

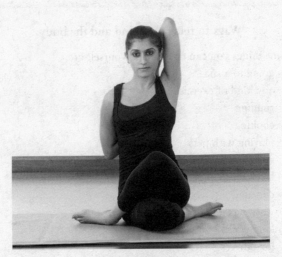

Goumukhasana

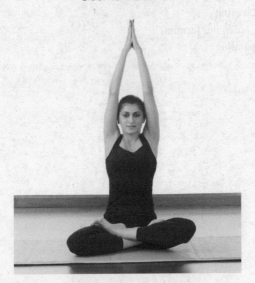

Parvatasana in Padmasana

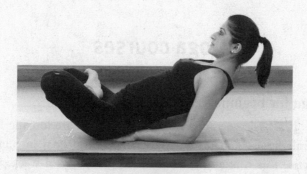

Tolangulasana

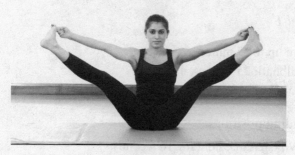

Merudandasana

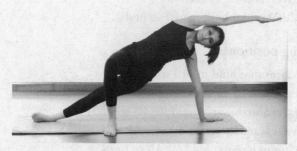

Saral Santolanasana

Yoga courses

Yoga for beginners

This is a basic yoga course for novices who are looking for overall fitness and do not have any special goal in mind. Practise this routine for three months, six days a week, till you can do all exercises well and comfortably. You can then progress to level 2.

Level 1

Warm up for 5 minutes
Kapalbhati: 25 strokes, 4 rounds
Suryanamaskars: 10 rounds

Standing positions:

1. Vrikshasana: hold for 10 seconds
2. Tadasana: hold for 10 seconds
3. Trikonasana: 10 seconds
4. Utkatasana: hold for 10 seconds

Sitting positions:

1. Vajrasana: hold for 10 seconds
2. Parvatasana in Padmasana: hold for 10 seconds
3. Janu Shirshasana: hold for 10 seconds
4. Vakrasana: hold for 10 seconds
5. Gomukhasana: hold for 10 seconds
6. Ek Pada Ugrasana: hold for 10 seconds

Supine positions:

1. Crocodile series 6 variations: hold for 10 seconds each
2. Saral Santolanasana with one leg forward and hand parallel to the ear: hold for 10 seconds each side, 1 set
3. Ardha Halasana: hold for 10 seconds
4. Pavanmuktasana: hold for 10 seconds
5. Setubandhasana: hold for 10 seconds
6. Naukasana: hold for 10 seconds
7. Vipreetkarni: hold for 10 seconds
8. Saral Matsyasana: hold for 10 seconds

Prone position

1. Niralambasana: hold for 10 seconds
2. Bhujangasana: hold for 10 seconds
3. Poorna Shalabhasana: hold for 10 seconds

Sitting positions in Sukhasana:

1. Kapalbhati kriya: 25 strokes, 5 rounds
2. Deep breathing: 5 seconds
3. Brahma Mudra: 3 rounds
4. Chandrabhedan Pranayam: 5 rounds
5. Suryabhedan Pranayam: 5 rounds
6. Anulom Vilom: 3 rounds
7. Om chanting or any auspicious chant: 3 rounds
8. Relaxation: 5 minutes
9. Meditation: sit calmly and quietly for 2 minutes

Yoga for elementary yoga practitioners

This is a general course for people who have followed the beginners' course for at least three months. You can move on to level 3 after you have followed this routine regularly for six days a week for six months. Before you get to the advanced level, you must feel the difference in your body, otherwise continue with the regime till you do so.

Level 2

Warm up for 5 minutes
Kapalbhati: 50 strokes, 4 rounds
1. Suryanamaskar (15 rounds, 1 set, take a break, then 10 rounds, 1 set) slowly = 25 rounds

Standing positions:

1. Padahastasana: hold for 10 seconds, 2 sets
2. Shishpadangustasana: hold for 10 seconds, 1 set
3. Garudasana: hold for 10 seconds each side, 1 set
4. Side bending Chakrasana: hold for 10 seconds, 2 sets

Sitting positions:

1. Ardha Matsyendrasana: hold for 10 seconds, each side, 2 sets
2. Paschimottanasana: hold for 10 seconds, 2 sets
3. SuptaVajrasana: hold for 10 seconds, 2 sets
4. Yog Mudra: hold for 10 seconds 1 set
5. Bhadrasana: hold for 10 seconds, 2 sets
6. Ustrasana: hold for 10 seconds, 1 set
7. Tolangulasana: hold for 10 seconds, 1 set

Supine positions:

1. Vipreetkarni: hold for 10 seconds, 2 sets
2. Sarvangasana: hold for 10 seconds, 2 sets
3. Matsyasana: hold for 10 seconds, 2 sets
4. Poorna Halasana: hold for 10 seconds, 2 sets

Prone positions:

1. Sarpasana: hold for 10 seconds, 2 sets
2. Naukasana: hold 10 seconds, 2 sets
3. Dhanurasana: hold 10 seconds, 2 sets

Sitting positions:

1. Brahma Mudra: 3 rounds
2. Sheetali Pranayam: 5 to 10 rounds
3. Ujjayi Pranayam: 5 to 10 rounds while exhaling
4. Bhramari Pranayam: 5 to 10 rounds
5. Om chanting or any auspicious chant: 5 rounds
6. Meditation: sit for 5 minutes calmly and quietly

Yoga for advanced yoga practitioners

This is a general course for people who have mastered the exercises in level 1 and level 2. These exercises are not simple and will require an enhanced level of fitness especially flexibility and endurance.

Level 3

Warm up for 5 minutes
1. Suryanamaskar: 50 rounds slowly (Karnapeedasana: 30 seconds and Chakrasana: 15 seconds)

Standing positions:

1. Vrikshasana: hold on right and left side for 30 seconds each, 2 sets
2. Pada Hastasana: hold for 30 seconds, 2 sets
3. Garudasana: hold on right and left side for 30 seconds each, 2 sets.
4. Utkatasana: hold on right and left side for 30 seconds each, 2 sets
5. Ardha Chandrasana: hold on right and left side for 30 seconds each, 2 sets

Sitting positions:

1. Ardha Matsyendrasana: hold on right and left side for 30 seconds each, 2 sets
2. Paschimottanasana: hold for 30 seconds, 2 sets
3. Ek Pada Vygrahasana: hold on right and left side for 30 seconds each, 2 sets
4. Akarna Dhanurasana: hold on right and left side for 30 seconds each, 2 sets
5. Ustrasana: hold for 30 seconds, 2 sets
6. Ugrasana: hold for 30 seconds, 2 sets
7. Padmasana: hold for 30 seconds, 2 sets
8. Vajrasana: hold for 30 seconds, 2 sets
9. Baddha Padmasana: hold for 30 seconds, 2 sets
10. Kapotasana: hold for 30 seconds, 2 sets

Supine positions:

1. Shavasana: 2 minutes
2. Sarvanganasana: hold for 30 seconds, 1 set

3. Matsyasana: hold for 20 seconds, 1 set
4. Poorna Halasana: hold for 30 seconds, 1 set

Prone positions:

1. Sarpasana: hold for 30 seconds, 2 sets
2. Poorna Shalabhasana: hold for 20 seconds, 2 sets
3. Naukasana: hold for 30 seconds, 2 sets
4. Dhanurasana: hold for 30 seconds, 2 sets
5. Makarasana: hold for 1 minute
6. Brahma Mudra: 3 rounds
7. Simhasana: 5 rounds
8. Kapalbhati: 100 strokes, 5 rounds
9. Bhastrika: 5 rounds
10. Ujjayi Pranayam: 10 rounds
11. Anulom Vilom: 10 rounds
12. Bhramari Pranayam: 10 rounds
13. Om recitation or any other auspicious chant: 10 rounds
14. Breath consciousness in Shavasana: 2 minutes

Directions for exercises

1. *Akarna Dhanurasana:* Sit on the floor stretching both legs together in front, hands by the side, and palms resting on the floor. Now bend forward to hold the big toe of your right leg with the help of the forefinger and thumb of your right hand. Similarly hold the big toe of the left leg with the forefinger and thumb of the left hand; then pull the right leg back till the toe touches the right ear. Hold for some time breathing normally, and come back to the original position. Repeat the same with the other leg.

2. *Anulom Vilom Pranayam:* Use the thumb of your right hand to close your right nostril and inhale with your left nostril. Then close your left nostril with your right hand's index and middle fingers and exhale from the right nostril. Now, in the reverse manner, inhale with the right nostril, close your right nostril with your right hand's thumb then exhale with the left. This forms one round of Anulom Vilom Pranayam. (see p. 68)

3. *Ardha Baddha Padmottanasana:* Stand with both feet together. Bending the right knee hold your ankle with your hand, balancing the body on the left leg. Place the right foot on the left thigh. Raise the hands up with the palms facing each other in Namaskar Mudra. Hold this position for some time, breathing normally and slowly come back to the original position. Repeat the same with the other leg. (see p. 161)

4. *Ardha Chandrasana* (standing position): Stand with both feet together, hands by the side and put your right leg forward. Bend your right knee at a 90-degree angle to the floor, pushing your left leg behind till you feel the stretch on your left thigh. Then inhale and raise your hands up in Namaskar Mudra, straighten the elbows, and arch your back. Hold for some time with normal breathing. Repeat the same with the other leg. (see p. 67)

5. *Ardha Halasana:* Lie in a supine position with legs together, hands by the side of the body, palms resting on the floor. Now while exhaling, raise both legs together gradually up to 30, 45, 60 and 90 degree angles. Hold each angle for 10 counts, with normal breathing, then slowly inhale and come down from 90 to 60, 45 and 30 degree angles respectively.

6. *Ardha Kapotasana:* Sit on your knees in Vajrasana. Now get up on your knees, and put the right leg forward. Now bend your upper body with the palms resting on the floor. Then bend your right knee putting it on the floor, stretching the left leg behind with the knee straight and toes facing outwards. Now balance the body in the Namaskar position. Inhale and raise the hands upwards and hold for some time, breathing normally. Come back slowly to the original position. Repeat the same with the other side. (see p. 233)

7. *Ardha Matsyendrasana:* Sit on the floor with both the legs extended together, hands by the side of the body, and palms resting on the floor. Now bend the right leg at the knee, and slowly put the right heel at the perineum. Then, bending the left leg, bring it from above the right

knee and place it by the side, on the floor. The knee of the left leg should face the ceiling. Now bring the right hand on the left side, over the left knee and hold your left ankle with your right hand. Twisting the body to the left side, look backwards, and place the left hand on the floor close to your spine with the elbow straightened. Hold for some time, breathing normally, and come back slowly to the original position. Repeat the same with the other side and the other leg. (see p. 60)

8. *Ardha Naukasana:* Lie down on your back with your feet together and your palms resting on your thighs. Inhale slowly and raise one leg up, simultaneously raising the upper body and hands upwards, towards the toe. Hold for some time while breathing normally. Then come down slowly to the original position and repeat with the other leg. (see p. 118)

9. *Ardha Padma Padottanasana:* Sit stretching both the legs together in front, hands by the side, palms resting on the floor. Now bend your right knee and place the right foot (ankle) on top of your left thigh. Next, bend the left knee and hold the left ankle with your hands and raise the left leg upward and straighten the knee. Balance on the back of your buttocks, and bring the left leg closer to the body. Hold for some time, with normal breathing. Then come down to the original position and repeat the same with the other leg.

10. *Ardha Pavanmuktasana:* Lie in a supine position with legs together, hands by the side, and palms resting on the floor. Bend right leg slowly towards your chest, hold your right knee and press it well towards the chest.

Then while exhaling, raise the chin up and try to touch the right knee, hold this for some time while breathing normally. Then come back to the original position and repeat the same with the other leg.

11. *Ardha Shalabhasana:* Lie in a prone position and bring your legs together, toes pointing outward, hands by the side of the body, fists closed, and forehead touching the floor. Then slowly raise the right leg without bending at the knee. Do not tilt the pelvis. Hold for some time with normal breathing, come back to the original position, and repeat the same with the other leg.

12. *Ardha Triyak Naukasana:* Lie down on your back with your feet together and your palms resting on your thighs. Inhale slowly and raise one leg up. Raise the upper body upwards while twisting towards the opposite side. Now place your right hand behind your head and hold for some time while breathing normally. Come down slowly to the original position and repeat the same with the other leg. (see p. 118)

13. *Baddha Padmasana:* Sit with both legs stretched out together in front, hands by the side, and palms resting on the floor. Now bend the right leg at the knee and put the right ankle on the left thigh, knee downwards. Bend the left leg at the knee and put the left ankle on the right thigh, knee downwards, both knees touching the floor. Then take your right hand to the left side and left hand to the right side from behind and hold the right toe with the right hand and left toe with the left hand, while keeping your back straight. Hold this for some time, breathing normally,

then release the toes and the legs and come back to the original position.

14. *Bhadrasana:* Sit on the floor with your legs extended in front of you, hands by the side, and back straight. Now slowly bend your knees downwards while placing the soles of your feet together. Hold your toes with the hands, and slowly move your knees up and down a few time to loosen the muscles of your inner thighs. Then hold your feet with both hands and push your knees towards the floor. Hold for some time breathing normally and then slowly come back to the original position. (see p. 159)

15. *Bhastrika Pranayam:* Sit in any meditative or comfortable position on the floor, with the back straight and shoulder muscles relaxed. Do 25 strokes of Kapalbhati and proceed to one round of Anulom Vilom without any break. This is one round of Bhastrika.

16. *Bhramri Pranayam:* Sit in any meditative or comfortable position on the floor, with your back straight, shoulder muscles relaxed, and eyes closed. Inhale deeply and exhale slowly while making a sound like that of a bee, without giving stress to the throat and facial muscles.

17. *Bhujangasana:* Lie in a prone position, legs together, toes together and pointing outwards, hands by the side of the body, palms facing upwards, and forehead on the floor. Now bend hands from the elbows, place the palms on the floor near each side of the shoulder. The thumb should be under the armpit. Inhale and raise your chin, turn your head upwards as much as possible, and raise your upper body up to the navel. Try to keep the palms off the floor by tucking the elbows close to the body. Hold this for

some time breathing normally, then while exhaling come
down to the original position. (see p. 65)

18. *Brahma Mudra:* Sit in Padmasana in Gyan Mudra
    (index finger touching the tip of thumb). Now slowly
    turn your neck towards the right side and hold for 5
    seconds, then repeat the process with the other side and
    hold again for 5 seconds. Now bring your neck back
    to the original position and raise your chin up. Hold it
    there for 5 seconds, then slowly bring your neck down
    and hold it there for 5 seconds and come back to the
    original position.

19. *Chakrasana:* Lie in a supine position, legs together,
    hands by the side, palms facing the floor. Now bend
    your legs at the knees, and place your feet apart on
    the floor close to the butt. Place your hands under the
    shoulder, palms facing down, and elbows upwards.
    Slowly lift the waist and upper body upwards with
    the help of the hands, while keeping the neck muscles
    relaxed. Hold this for some time breathing normally.
    While coming back first bend the elbows, put the head
    on the floor, then shoulder, upper back, mid-back,
    lower back, and finally place the butt on the floor and
    come back to the original position. (see p. 61)

20. *Chakrasana* (side bending): While standing, put your
    feet together with the hands on the side. Now raise
    your right hand up and stretch while bending your
    body towards the left side. Hold for some time, and
    come back to the original position. Repeat it with the
    other side. (see p. 161)

21. *Chandrabedhan Pranayam:* Sit in any meditative

or comfortable position on the floor, with the eyes closed, back straight, and shoulders relaxed. With the thumb of your right hand close the right nostril, and inhale from the left nostril. Then close the left nostril with the index and middle fingers of your right hand, and exhale from the right nostril. This completes Chandrabedhan Pranayam.

22. *Chandranamaskar*: Also known as Ardha Chandrasana, it is supposed to be done in between position positions 4 and 5, and between positions 9 and 10 of Suryanamaskar. Take your hands upwards in Namaskar Mudra and hold it there, breathing normally.

23. *Dhanurasana*: Lie in a prone position facing the floor, feet together, hands by the side and forehead on the floor. Now bend your knees, hold the ankles with both hands and, while inhaling, raise the upper body and legs up together. Hold for some time, breathing normally and come back to the original position. (see p. 66)

24. *Dwi Pada Uttan Paschimottanasana*: Sit on the floor with the legs straight in the front, hands by the side of the body and palms resting on the floor. Slowly bend the legs from the knees, hold the right toe with the right hand's middle and index finger, and the left toe with the left hand's middle and index fingers. Now try to raise both the legs up while balancing the body on the middle part of the buttocks, keeping the knees straight. Hold this position, breathing normally, then slowly come back to the starting position. (see p. 150)

25. *Ek Padasana*: This asana is done in the standing position. Put your feet together, and hands by the side. Place your

palms together in the Namaskar position and raise your hands up. Now bend forward and simultaneously raise the right leg up straight, without bending the left leg making a T shape. Hold for some time with each leg, breathing normally.

26. *Ek Padasana* variation (interlocking the hand behind your back) in standing position: Place your legs together and your hands by the side. Slowly take your hands to the back, from the sides. Interlocking your fingers with each other, fix your palms and inhale. Stretch your hands behind, bending your upper body forward raise your right leg up and make a 90-degree angle to the floor. Hold for some time breathing normally. (see p. 114)

27. *Ek Pada Ardha Halasana:* Lie in a supine position with your legs together, and hands by the side. While exahaling, raise the right leg upto 60 degrees from the floor then inhale and come back. Repeat the same with the left leg. Keep repeating this with alternate legs for some time.

28. *Ek Pada Ardha Halasana variation:* Lie on your back on the floor. Keep your hands straight at the shoulder level, with palms resting on the floor. Raise your right leg at a 90-degree angle to the floor. Turn your leg towards the right side of the floor, till you feel a contraction in your inner thighs. Hold for 20 seconds. Turn towards the left side of the floor till you get a contraction on your outer thighs. Hold for some time. Keep changing the leg position in the same way upto 20 to 30 times.

29. *Ek Pada Hasta Santolanasana* (hand and leg upwards): Sit in cat pose, straighten your knees, move the shoulders

forward and the buttock downwards until the body is
straight like in position no. 5 of SuryaNamaskar. Now
turn the body to the right side and balance the body on
the elbow and the forearm (keep the other foot on top of
the lower foot). Now raise the hand parallel to the ear.
Hold it for some time breathing normally. Then slowly
repeat the same with the other side.

30. *Ek Padottanasana*: Sit straight and stretch both legs
forward, hands by the side, with palms resting on the
floor. Now bend the right knee and place the foot flat on
the floor in front of the right buttock. Bend the left leg
keeping the knee on the floor and place the heel close to
your pelvic area. Now hold the toes of the right leg with
your hands and straighten the knee while raising the
leg upwards. Try to touch your nose with knee keeping
your back straight. Hold this for some time breathing
normally and come back slowly to the original position.
Repeat the same with the other leg.

31. *Ek Pada Ugrasana*: Sit straight on the floor, stretching
both the legs together in front of you with palms resting
on the floor. Now slowly widen the legs, as much as you
can bending slightly forward. Bend your right leg at the
knee with the help of your right hand, pushing your right
foot under your left thigh. Now slowly raise your hands
upwards, bend forward and try to hold your big toe, pulling
it towards you. Try to straighten your back as much as you
can. Hold this position for some time, breathing normally.
Slowly come back to the starting position and repeat the
process with the other leg. (see p. 159)

32. *Ek Pada Uttan Angusthasana*: Slowly come back to the

starting position. Stand straight with your feet together and hands by the sides. Now slowly bend the right knee while balancing the body on the left leg. Hold the toe of the right leg with the right hand and the middle and the index fingers. Then slowly turn the right leg towards the right side and stretch the leg till the knee is straight. Raise the left hand upwards, parallel to the ear. Hold this posture, breathing normally. Come back to the normal position and then repeat with the other side. (see coloured insert pages)

33. *Ek Pada Uttan Paschimottanasana*: Sit on the floor with the legs straight in the front, hands by the side of the body, and palms resting on the floor. Now bend the right knee and hold the right ankle with both hands, keeping the right knee straight while raising it up as much as you can. Keep your back straight and hold it there, breathing normally. Now slowly come back to the normal position and repeat the process with the other leg. (see p. 150)

34. *Ek Pada Vyaghrasana*: Sit on the floor with palms resting on the floor and your knees touching the ground like in cat pose. Place your hands under your shoulders. Your knees should be apart in the same level. Now raise your right leg upwards without applying pressure on your back. Bend your right leg at the knee, taking your right hand behind trying to hold your right foot. Now while holding your right foot, raise your head backwards and raise your right leg further, as much as you can. Hold this position, breathing normally. Slowly come back to the starting position. Repeat the posture with the other leg. (see p. 160)

35. *Garudasana:* This asana is done in the standing position.
     With your feet together, and hands by the side. Bend
     your knees slightly, and entangle your right leg over the
     left leg. Similarly, entangle your right hand with your left
     hand and bring it to the chest level balancing the body on
     one leg. Hold for some time breathing normally. Follow
     the same with the other leg and hand. (see p. 231)

36. *Gomukhasana:* Sit on the floor stretching your legs
     forward. Bend both your knees slightly. Place your left
     leg under your right thigh and take your right leg over
     your left leg, making sure both your knees are under
     each other. Now take your right hand with elbow facing
     the ceiling behind your back with your fingers facing
     downwards. Now take your left hand behind your back.
     Try holding both your palms together, making sure
     your entire back is straight and aligned with your neck.
     Breathe normally once you are in this posture. Repeat
     the same with the other leg and hand. Hold for some
     time and come back to the original position.

37. *Hanumanasana:* Stand straight with feet together and
     hands by the side. Spread your legs apart slowly as much
     as you can, and turn both your feet and your upper body
     towards the right side. Inhale slowly while raising both
     your hands up with the palms facing each other. In the
     final position, make sure both the knees are straight,
     palms are together the head tilted upwards while your
     back is arched. Hold for sometime, breathing normally
     and slowly come back to the normal position. Repeat
     the same with the other side. (see coloured insert pages)

38. *Jalandar Bandha* (can be done while inhaling and

exhaling): Sit in any meditative or comfortable position on the floor with your back straight and shoulders relaxed. Inhale slowly, hold your breath, and gradually drop your chin down as much as you can. Hold for as long as you can. Now slowly get your chin back to the original position and exhale through your nose. Sit in any meditative or comfortable position on the floor with your back straight and shoulders relaxed. Inhale slowly through your nose and exhale holding your breath out. Drop your chin down as much as you can and hold for as long as you can. Lift your chin back gradually to the original position and inhale slowly through your nose.

39. *Janu Shirshasana:* Sit on the floor with both legs stretched in front, keeping the back straight and the hands by the side. Bend your right knee and place your right foot on the inner thigh of the left leg. Inhale and raise both hands upwards, and then exhale slowly bending forward and hold the ankle of the right leg. Try and place your forehead on the knee and try and touch the elbow to the floor. Hold it there for some time, breathing normally. Repeat the same with the other leg. (see coloured insert pages)

40. *Jumping Jack:* Stand straight normally. Now jump forward with your feet apart at about a distance of one foot. Then jump back to the normal position. Keep breathing normally.

41. *Kati Chakrasana* crocodile series 1: Lie in the supine position, with both legs together and palms resting on the floor. Then spread your arms shoulder level apart and bend your right knee, putting the right foot on the left thigh. Right knee facing upwards; slowly bring your

right knee towards the left side while twisting your back towards the right side and neck to the opposite side. Hold for some time, breathing normally, and come back to the original position. Repeat the same on the other side.

42. *Kati Chakrasana* crocodile series 2: Lie in the supine position, with both legs together and palms resting on the floor. Spread the arms apart in the same distance as between the shoulders, with palms resting on the floor. Now bend your right knee, placing the right foot on the left thigh with the right knee facing upwards. Slowly bring your right knee towards the left side while twisting your back towards the right side and neck to the opposite side. Hold the position, breathing normally. Come back to the starting position and repeat the process with the other side.

43. *Kati Chakrasana* crocodile series 3: Lie in the supine position, with both legs together and palms resting on the floor. Spread the arms apart in the same distance as between the shoulders, with palms resting on the floor. Now raise the right leg and put the right heel in between the big and the small toe of the left leg while twisting your back towards the left side. Try to touch the floor with the right toe towards the left side, making the neck face the opposite side. Hold this position, breathing normally. Come back to the starting position and repeat the same process on the other side.

44. *Kati Chakrasana* crocodile series 4: Lie in the supine position, with both legs together and palms resting on the floor. Spread the arms apart in the same distance as between the shoulders, with palms resting on the floor.

Bend your right knee, placing the right foot on the left shin (below the knee) and the right knee facing upwards. Slowly bring your right knee towards the left side while twisting your back towards the right side and neck to the opposite side. Hold this position for some time, breathing normally. Come back to the starting position slowly and repeat the process on the other side.

45. *Kati Chakrasana* crocodile series 5: Lie in the supine position, with both legs together and palms resting on the floor. Spread the arms apart in the same distance as between the shoulders, with palms resting on the floor. Now bend both the knees together facing upwards, then slowly bring the knees towards the left side while twisting the back and turning the neck to the right side. Hold it in this position, breathing normally. Slowly come back to the starting position and repeat the same on the other side.

46. *Kati Chakrasana* crocodile series 6: Lie in the supine position, with both legs together and palms resting on the floor. Spread the arms apart in the same distance as between the shoulders, with palms resting on the floor. Now raise the right leg at an angle of 90 degrees from the floor and slowly bring the right foot towards the left side on the floor without bending the right knee but twisting the back and turning the neck to the right side. Hold this position, breathing normally, then come back to the starting position. Repeat process with the other side.

47. *Konasana:* Stand straight with your legs together and hands on the side. Now widen your legs sideways and

spread your arms shoulder level. Slowly bend your upper body towards the right. Keep the knees straight while trying to hold the ankle of the right leg, taking the left hand towards the ceiling. Hold tight for some time breathing normally and slowly come back to the original position. Repeat the same with the other side.

48. *Jalneti kriya:* You need to do this near a washbasin or someplace where you brush your teeth. Add a pinch of salt in a glass of lukewarm water and mix it properly. Transfer the water to the Jalneti pot. Bend forward in a 90-degree angle from the floor, then turn your neck towards the left side and open your mouth to inhale and exhale. Now with the Jalneti pipe, let the water enter your left nostril and allow it to come through the other nostril while breathing from the mouth. Continue to do this till the Jalneti pot is empty. After you have completed this process, do 30 strokes of Kapalbhatis in standing position, facing the washbasin to clean your nostril. Perform the same procedure with the other nostril.

49. *Makarasana* (relaxative pose): Lie in prone position, feet together, hands by the side, palms facing upwards and forehead touching the floor. Now spread the legs apart and turn the toes sideways, then stretch the hands forward. Place the right hand under the left armpit, and left hand on the right shoulder making sure one elbow is under the other. Relax in this position breathing normally.

50. *Marjariasana* (cat pose): Sit on the floor with your palms resting on the floor like a cat. Place your hands under your shoulders. Your knees should be apart in the

same level. Now inhale while raising the head upwards and pushing the back downwards, and make a major contraction on your butt muscles. Hold for some time. Exhale while lowering the head and stretching the spine upwards. The head will now be in between the arms facing the thighs. Hold this position for some time and slowly come back to the original position.

51. *Matsyasana* (fish pose): Sit in Padmasana. Taking your elbow's support, lie on your back slowly. Now bend your head backwards and touch it o the ground, while stretching your mid-back. Hold your toes with your index finger and keep the elbows on the ground at the same time. Hold for some time, breathing normally and come back to the original position. (see p. 197)

52. *Merudandasana:* Sit straight on the floor, with your legs stretched out together, hands by the side, and palms resting on the floor. Now widen the legs apart as much as you can, and slowly bend forward. Hold the right big toe with the right hand and the left big toe with the left hand. Now slowly stretch the legs upwards while leaning the body backwards and balancing it on the tailbone and hips, with the arms straight. Balance for some time, breathing normally, and then slowly come back to the original position. (see p. 259)

53. *Natrajasana:* Stand straight with your feet together, and hands by the side of your thighs. Bend the right knee, holding the ankle with the right hand behind the body. Balance on the left leg and make sure that the knee of the left leg is straight. Now raise your left hand in front of you. Raise and stretch the right leg backwards

slowly, as high as you can, making sure that the right hip is not twisted and the leg is raised directly behind the body. Hold this for some time in a comfortable position, breathing normally, and slowly come back to the original position. (see p. 67)

54. *Naukasana* (on the back): Lie down on your back with your feet together and your palms resting on your thighs. Inhale and raise both legs up, then raise the upper body off the floor. Hold for some time while breathing normally keeping your hands parallel to the floor. Return to the original position slowly. (see p. 66)

55. *Naukasana* (on the stomach): Lie down on the stomach with feet together, hands by the sides of the body, palms resting on the floor. Slowly bring both your hands parallel to your ears, making sure that the feet are together and the toes facing outwards. Now, slowly inhale and raise your upper and lower body together at the same time, making sure the hands keep touching the ears at all times. Once your body is in this boat like posture, hold it there and breathe normally. Slowly come back to the starting position.

56. *Naukasana* variation 1 (hands across the chest): Lie on your back, feet together, and palms resting on your thighs. Inhale slowly and raise both legs up, folding your arms across your chest. Hold for some time, while breathing normally, and slowly come down to the original position. (see p. 116)

57. *Naukasana* variation 2 (hands parallel to the ears): Lie on your back, feet together and palms resting on your thighs. Inhale slowly and raise both legs up, raising your arms parallel to your ears. Hold for some time

while breathing normally and slowly come down to the original position. (see p. 117)

58. *Niralambasana:* Lie in a prone position with your forehead on the floor, hands by the side, legs together, and toes pointed outwards. Slowly stretch the arms forward, and bend the elbows raising the head upwards. Place the chin on the palms, with your fingers touching the cheeks, making sure the elbows are together. Hold this for some time breathing normally. Then slowly come back to the original position.

59. *Pada Hastasana:* Standing straight with your legs together, hands by the side, and palms facing inside. Now inhale, raising the hands upwards, stretch the body. Then exhale slowly and bend forward touching the floor, or toes, with the hands without bending the knees in the final position. Drop neck slowly and hold for some time breathing normally. Inhale slowly and come back to the original position.

60. *Pada Prasar Paschimottanasana* (sideways): Sit on the floor with the legs together in front, hands by the side, and palms resting on the floor. Slowly widen the legs as far as you can. Put your hands behind, interlock the fingers, and slowly turn the body towards the right leg. Inhale slowly and bend forward while stretching the hands behind, and try to touch the forehead to the right knee. Hold this position for some time while breathing normally. Then come back slowly to the original position while inhaling. Repeat the same with the other side.

Do not try hard to reach the final position if you can't. Perform this asana slowly and gradually.

61. *Padmasana:* Sit on the floor and stretch the legs forward. Place the palms on the side of the body. Now, holding the sole of the right foot, place it on the left thigh and holding the sole of the left foot, place it on the right thigh. Keeping the back straight place the palms on the knees in Gyan Mudra. Close your eyes slowly and focus on your normal breath. Hold for some time and come back slowly to the original position. (see p. 231)

62. *Parighasana:* Sit in Vajrasana with your hands on the knees. Now stand slowly on the knees, and stretch the right leg to the right side keeping the knee straight. Inhale and raise your hands upwards, and while exhaling, bend the body to the right side and try to hold the right ankle with both hands. Hold for some time breathing normally, and come back slowly to the original position and repeat the same with the other leg and side. (see p. 160)

63. *Parivritta Janu Shirshasana:* Sit erect with both legs together in front, hands by the side of the body, and palms on the floor. Widen the legs apart and bend the left leg at the knee, putting the left heel against the perineum. Now hold the right leg with the right hand. Inhale, and raise the left hand upwards, and exhale slowly. Bending the upper body sideways towards the right side, try to catch the right toe with the left hand. Hold this for some time, breathing normally, and come back to the original position. Repeat the same with the other side.

64. *Parvatasana:* See Suryanamaskar.

65. *Parvatasana* in *Padmasana:* Sit straight in Padmasana with palms resting on the floor. Get the palms together, facing each other, in Namaskar Mudra close to the chest.

Inhale slowly and raise your hands upwards and stretch your arms as much as you can without exerting pressure on the neck. Breathe normally and hold for some time. Slowly come back to the original position. (see p. 258)

66. *Paschimottanasana:* Sit on the floor, and your legs straight and palms on your thighs, keeping your heels on the floor. Inhale and take your hands upwards with your palms facing each other. Now bend forward and try to hold your foot with the help of your hands, without bending your knees. Keep bending forward as much as you can, while trying to touch your knees with your nose. Hold this for some time breathing normally and then slowly come back to the original position. Initially, one may not be flexible enough to get into this posture as the fat in the abdomen may act as a barrier. Nonetheless, at the initial stage bend as much as you can, but don't bend your knees. Don't do it too fast, as it is more important to remain in the bending posture for a longer duration than doing it more number of times. (see p. 148)

67. *Pavanmuktasana:* Lie in supine position with your legs together, hands by the side, and palms resting on the floor. Slowly bend both knees together towards the chest. Hold your knees with your hands and pull well towards the chest. Raise your chin up between the knees, and hold and for some time, breathing normally. Then come back to the original position.

68. *Poorna Halasana:* Lie on you back with feet together, hands by the side and palms resting on the floor. Inhale, and then while exhaling raise both your legs up. With

the help of your palms, raise your hip up and bring your toes above your head, without bending your knees. Now interlock your fingers with each other, stretch your arms together and hold the position. Breathe normally while in this position, keeping the neck and facial muscles relaxed. Follow the positions in reverse order to come back to the original position. (see p. 61)

69. *Poorna Shalabhasana:* Lie in the prone position, bring the legs together, toes pointing outwards, hands by the side of the body, fists closed, and chin on the floor. Then raise both the legs slowly without bending at the knee. Do not tilt the pelvis. Hold this for some time with normal breathing, and come back down slowly. (see p. 65)

70. *Poorna Triyak Naukasana:* Lie on your back with your feet together and your palms resting on your thighs. Inhale slowly and raise both legs up. Then raise the upper body and hands upwards towards your toes. Now turn your full body towards the right side of your right hip. Hold for some time and come back to the original position. Repeat the same with the other side. (see p. 117)

71. *Sahaj Pranayam:* Sit in any meditative or comfortable posture. Keep the back straight, shoulder, and elbow muscles relaxed and palms resting on the knees. Now, with the eyes closed inhale slowly and deeply from the nose and exhale from the nose as well. In this Pranayam focus on the breath without exerting the body and try to keep the number of inhalation and exhalations as same.

72. *Santolanasana* variation 1: Sit in the cat pose, straighten your knees, move the shoulders forward, and drop the

buttock until the body is straight like position no. 5 of Suryanamaskar. Hold as long as you can breathing normally. (see p. 114)

73. *Santolanasana* variation 2 (with one hand upwards): Sit in the cat pose, straighten your knees move the shoulders forward and the buttock downwards until the body is parallel to the floor. Turn your full body to the right side slowly and raise your left hand up to the shoulders' level. Make sure your upper body weight is on your right hand and lower body weight on both legs. Then come back to the original position. Repeat the same with the other side. Hold for some time, breathing normally. (see p. 115)

74. *Santolanasana* variation 3 (hand behind the back): Sit in a cat pose, straighten your knees move the shoulders forward and the buttock downwards until the body is straight like a position no. 5 of Suryanamaskar. Now turn the body to the right side and balance it on one hand taking the other hand behind the back and pushing the shoulder towards the ceiling. Hold for some time while breathing normally. Then slowly repeat with the other side. (see p. 115)

75. *Saral Santolanasana*: Sit in cat pose. Now straighten your knees, move your shoulders forward and press the buttock downwards until the body is straight like in position 5 of Suryanamaskar. Now turn the body to the left side and balance the body on the left hand and the left leg. Now place the right leg forward on the floor, making sure your right foot is in front of the left knee. Now raise the right hand parallel to the right ear. Hold

the position, breathing normally. Now come back to the starting position and repeat the process with the other side. (see p. 259)

76. *Sarpasana:* Lie on your stomach with your forehead touching the floor, hands by the side of your body, and palms by the side. Bend both your elbows slowly bringing your palms close to the chest, with elbows facing upwards close to your body. Inhale slowly raising your head, shoulders, chest, and stomach till your navel region, with the help of your hands. In the final position, hold for some time, breathing normally and then slowly come down to the original position. (see p. 89)

77. *Sarvangasana:* Lie down in the supine position with the legs together, hands by the side and palms facing the floor. Inhale slowly and while exhaling, raise both the legs together at a 90-degree angle to the floor. Now press the palms and bring the legs towards the head, so that the buttock faces upwards. Now bend the elbows and support the back with the palms. Then take the legs upwards till the legs, abdomen, and chest form a straight line. The chin should be placed against the jugular notch. Hold this for some time, breathing normally. While coming back to the original position first lower the buttocks, release the hands slowly and bring the legs down without raising the head. (see p. 197)

78. *Setubandhasana:* Lie on your back, and bend your knees. Keep your feet close to your hips with hands by the side, and palms resting on the floor. Inhale slowly and push the waist upwards as much as you can without any pressure on your neck. Hold for some time while

breathing normally.

79. *Setubandhasana* variation (with legs straight): Sit on the floor with the legs straight, hands by the side and palms resting on the floor. Now take your hands behind at a distance of about half a foot from the body with elbows straight, palms resting on the floor and fingers facing inside. Now inhale and raise the body from the waist, keeping the legs straight. Try to keep the toes on the floor without lifting the heel and slowly drop the neck behind with the chin facing upwards towards the ceiling. Hold this position, breathing normally. While exhaling, slowly come back to the starting position.

80. *Sharnagat Mudra*: Sit in Vajrasana with the back straight. Slowly inhale and raise both the hands upwards. Now exhale, and bend forward slowly. Touch your palms on the floor by stretching the arms but without bending the elbows. Now place your head on the floor with the abdomen pressed to the thighs. Do not raise the buttocks. Hold this position.

81. *Shavasana:* Lie down on the back with the legs together and hands by the side. Spread the legs apart slowly, keeping the heels inside and toes outside. Keep your hands away from the body, with the palms facing upwards. Close your eyes, loosen, and relax all the muscles in the body and focus on your normal and natural breathing.

82. *Sheetali Pranayam:* Sit in any meditative or comfortable position. Close your eyes and relax your whole body with normal breathing. Put the tongue on the lower lip and try to roll the tongue. Inhale deeply from the mouth and slowly close the mouth and exhale through the nose.

This is one round of Sheetali Pranayama.

83. *Sheetkari Pranayam* (benefits are the same so those who can't roll their tongue as required in Sheetali Pranayam can do this Pranayam): Sit in any meditative or comfortable posture on the floor. The back should be straight and shoulders relaxed with hands on the knees, fingers relaxed, and eyes closed. Now put the lower and upper teeth together and fix the tongue between the gap of the teeth. Then separate the lips while showing the teeth. Inhale from the mouth and exhale from the nose. This is one round of Sheetkari Pranayam.

84. *Shirsh Pada Angusthanasana*: Stand straight with both the feet together and hands by the side. Slowly, widen the legs sideways as much as possible with toes pointing outwards. Bend the right leg at the knee at a 90-degree angle to the floor. Then take the hands behind, interlocking the fingers while inhaling. Next while exhaling, bend the body forward towards the right foot, and try to touch the forehead to the right toe, with hands stretched backwards and raised to the ceiling. Hold this for some time breathing normally. Then while inhaling come back to the original position. Repeat the same with the other side.

85. *Sideways Naukasana*: Lie down at 90 degrees with your weight on the right elbow and legs together in front. Now lift your upper body slowly. While exhaling lift your legs upwards. You can move your legs a little forward so that you can lift the legs comfortably till you are at 45 degrees from the floor. Hold the position, breathing normally. Slowly come back to the normal position and repeat the same on the other side.

86. *Simhasana*: Sit in Vajrasana on your knees and place your palms on it, taking care that your elbows are straight. Now, inhale slowly and while exhaling stretch your facial muscles by pulling out your tongue and pressing it downwards towards the chin. While you are doing this, make sure that you look between your eyebrows. Hold for 15 to 20 seconds, while breathing normally. Repeat it 3 to 5 times.

87. *Sukhasana*: Sit on the floor with legs crossed, keeping the entire body relaxed. Keep the back straight, and palms on the knees in Gyana Mudra keeping the eyes closed. Hold for some time breathing normally.

88. *Supta Tadasana*: Sit straight in Vajrasana, slowly keep the feet apart on the floor. Lean backwards on your right and left elbows. Now try and bend your head and back towards the floor as much as you can. Keep stretching till you are comfortable, the abdomen. Stretch the hands upwards and get the palms together in Namaskar Mudra. Hold for some time breathing normally. Now slowly, with the help of the elbows, come back to the original position. (see p. 149)

89. *Supta Vajrasana*: Sit straight in Vajrasan. Keep your feet apart on the floor. Lean backwards on your right and left elbows. Now try and bend your head and back towards the floor as much as you can till you are comfortable while stretching the abdomen. Keeping the hands on the thighs, hold for some time breathing normally. Now with the help of the elbows slowly come back to the original position. (see p. 149)

90. *Suryabhedan Pranayam*: Sit in any meditative or

comfortable posture. Close your left nostril with your index and middle fingers, and inhale with your right nostril. Close your right nostril with your right hand thumb and exhale through the left nostril.

91. *Suryanamaskar* (see p. 86 to 91)

Position 1 Namaskar Mudra: Stand straight with your feet together and hands by the side. Now bring your palms together close to your chest in Namaskar Mudra, breathing normally.

Position 2 back bending Chakrasana: Inhale and raise your hands upwards. Now arch your back and stretch your arms upwards as far back as you can. Once you are in this position, breathe normally.

Position 3 Padahastasana: Exhale and bend forward, touching your toes with your hands without bending the knees. Look downwards and breathe normally once you are in this posture.

Position 4 Ashwa Sanchalanasana: Place your palms on the floor while inhaling, bend the right leg between your hands at a 90-degree angle from the floor, then stretch the left leg backwards. Now arch your back and look upwards, breathing normally.

Position 5 Santolanasana: Exhale and place your right leg behind, so that it is in line with your left leg. Make sure your hands are aligned below with your shoulders. The shoulders, back, and hips should be in one straight line. Breathe normally when you are in this posture.

Position 6 Shashtanga Mudra: Bend the elbows, chin, chest and knees towards the floor. Tuck the elbows on the sides and close to the body. Now raise the hips upwards, breathing normally.

Position 7 Sarpasana: Inhale and raise the upper body on your elbows with the shoulders bending backwards and the chin upwards. The waist should touch the floor. Once in the final posture, breathe normally.

Position 8 Parvatasana: Exhale and raise the hips upwards, pushing the upper body behind and touching the heels on the floor. Keep your knees straight and neck facing downwards looking at the navel region, once in posture breathe normally.

Position 9 Ashwa Sanchalanasana: Inhale while placing your left leg forward and in between the hands. Now arch your back, press the chin upwards, keeping the palms flat on the floor. Breathe normally once you are in this posture.

Position 10 Padahastasana: Bring your left leg forward towards your right leg, keeping the knees straight. Now with the palms touching the toe and the neck relaxed. Once you attain this posture, breathe normally.

Position 11 back bending Chakrasana: Bring your palms together, inhale and raise the hands and the upper body upwards while arching your back. Breathe normally once you attain this posture.

Position 12 Namaskar Mudra: Come back to the starting position slowly while exhaling.

92. *Tadasana:* Stand straight with your feet shoulder width apart, and your hands to the side of your body. Inhale slowly raising your hands upwards with your palms facing each other. Stretch your entire body while standing on your toes. In the final position hold for some time, breathing normally. Come down to the original position

slowly, while exhaling. (see p. 230)

93. *Trataka kriya:* Sit in any meditative or comfortable position in a dark room. Put a candle in front of you at a distance of about 2 feet, at eye level. Now keep looking at the flame of the candle with the facial muscles relaxed till you blink your eyes. Then close your eyes and relax in Shavasana for 10 minutes. In this kriya it is initially difficult to stare for a long time, but the more you practice, the more time will keep on increasing.

94. *Trikonasana:* Stand straight with your legs together and hands by the side of the thighs. Spread your legs apart slowly upto a distance of 2 to 3 feet. Slowly raise both the hands sideways at shoulder level with the palms facing the floor. Then bend forward towards the right side, touching the big toe of the right leg with the left hand without bending the knees. Raise your right hand up and look up towards it, breathing normally. Hold this for some time and come back to the original position. Repeat the same with the other side. (see p. 148)

95. *Triyak Bhujangasana:* Lie in a prone position, with your legs together, toes together and pointing outwards, hands by the side of the body, palms facing upwards and forhead on the floor. Now bend hands from the elbows and place palms on the floor, near each side of the shoulder. The thumb should be under the armpit. Then inhale and raise the chin and turn the head backwards over the right shoulder as much as possible, and raise up to the navel. Hold for some time breathing normally. Then while exhaling come down

to the original position. Repeat the same with the left side.

96. *Ugrasana:* Sit straight on the floor stretching both legs together, in front of you, with palms resting on the floor. Now slowly widen legs, as much as you can. Bend forward slightly and try to hold the big toe of the right leg with the right hand, and the left toe with the left hand. Now pull the toes inside slowly towards the body without bending the knees and elbows. Try to keep the back straight, breathing normally. Hold there for some time and slowly come back to the original position. (see p. 232)

97. *Ujjayi Pranayam:* Sit straight in any meditative or comfortable posture. Now inhale slowly and deeply the nose and while exhaling, contract the air passage and exhale slowly with a whispering sound.

98. *Ustrasana:* Sit straight in Vajrasana. Slowly stand on the knees keeping them shoulder width apart. Now slowly turn the upper body to the right side and try to catch the right heel with the right hand, and the left heel with the left hand while balancing the body. After holding the heels, inhale and push the waist forward and drop the neck behind. Breath normally in the final position. Hold for some time. While exhaling come back to the normal position. (see p. 232)

99. *Utkatasana* (chair pose against the wall): Stand at a distance of 1½ feet from the wall. Place your back against the wall and bend your knees at a ninety degrees angle to the floor. Hold for some time while breathing normally.

100. *Utkatasana* (chair pose) level 1 and 2: Stand straight, feet

together, palms by the side of the body. Keep your feet apart, almost as much as the width of your shoulders. Now bend your knees at 90 degrees to the floor and slowly raise your hands in front of you at shoulder level. Stay in this posture for some time and breathe normally. Slowly come back to the starting position. This is level 2. Level 1 is for beginners, wherein you bend your knees not up to 90 degrees from the floor but as much as you can comfortably. (see p. 59)

101. *Utkatasana* (chair pose) level 3: Stand straight, feet together, palms by the side of the body. Keep your feet apart, almost as much as the width of your shoulders. Now bend your knees at 90 degrees to the floor. Slowly raise your heels, balancing the body on your toes. Now raise your hands in front at shoulder level. Hold this posture, breathing normally. (see p. 59)

102. *Uttanasana:* Stand straight with the hands on the side of the body. Now widen the legs as much as possible, toes facing outwards. Bend the legs at the knees with the knees facing outwards and hips below the hip joints. Keeping the back straight rest the palms on the floor and hold this for some time, breathing normally. Then come back to the original position. (see p. 162)

103. *Uttan Mandukasana:* Sit in Vajrasana. Now spread both the knees and make sure the toes are touching each other, keeping the back straight. Bend the right hand backwards from above the right shoulder and place the palm below the left shoulder. Now, bending the left hand, place the palm on the right shoulder.

Keeping the back and neck straight, breathe normally. Be in this position for some time. Come back slowly to the original position. (see p. 162)

104. *Vajrasana:* Sit with legs extended forward together, hands by the side of the body, and palms resting on the floor. Now bend the right leg at the knee and place the foot under the right buttock. Similarly bending the left leg, placing it under the left buttock. Hands should be resting on the thighs with the back straight. Hold for some time, then come back to the original position. (see p. 116)

105. *Vakrasana:* Sit straight on the floor, stretching the legs in front, hands by the side, and palms resting on the floor. Now slowly bend the right leg at the knee and place your right foot close to the left knee joint. With the right knee facing upwards now taking the right hand behind the palm on the floor close to the spine with the fingers facing upwards. Then take the left hand over the right knee and try to catch the right ankle, while twisting the head back towards the right side, and looking backwards. Breathing normally, hold for some time and come back to the original position. Repeat the same with the other side. (see p. 149)

106. *Vaman kriya:* You need to do this kriya near a wash basin or someplace where you brush your teeth. Add one tablespoonful of salt to one litre of lukewarm water. Drink all of it, as quickly as possible, until you feel you can't take any more. Now when your stomach is full, involuntarily you will feel like vomiting. Now, lean forwards, over the basin and insert the middle and index

fingers of your right hand, as deep as possible, into your
throat. Then vomit out all the water till you feel that
your stomach is empty. After this, relax in Shavasana for
10 minutes.

107. *Vipreetkarni:* Put your feet together and hands by the
sides with the palms resting on the floor. Now inhale
slowly and raise both your legs up, 90 degrees to the
floor. Then push your palms on the floor and raise your
hips up. Hold your waist with your hands in the final
position. Remember to keep your neck muscles relaxed
and breathe normally. Stay in this position for 15 to 20
seconds, then come back slowly to the original position
in a reverse manner. Follow it up with its counter pose,
Setubandhasana. (see p. 198)

108. *Vrikshasana* (tree pose): Stand straight with both feet
together and hands by the side. Now bend the right
leg at the knee and hold the right ankle with the right
hand. Place the right heel tight at the pelvic region,
while balancing the body on the left leg. Then get into
the Namaskar Mudra with palms together, close to
the chest. Balance this asana for some time breathing
normally. Come back slowly to the original position
and repeat the same with the other leg. (see p. 230)

109. *Yoga Mudra:* Sit in Padmasana with the back straight,
and hands by the side of the body. Now take the hands
behind the back and interlocking the fingers, inhale
slowly. Bend forward while exhaling and try to touch
the forehead to the floor while breathing normally.
Come back, while inhaling, to the original position.

Benefits of exercises

S. no	Asana	Area it works on	Benefits
1	Akarna Dhanurasana	hamstrings, arms, and the hip joint	• eases pain in the back and lumbar region • increases flexibility of thighs and shoulders • useful to those suffering from arthritis However, those suffering from frozen shoulder should not perform this asana.
2	Anulom Vilom Pranayam	all the systems inside the body	• purifies 72,000 nerves (nadis) in the body • balances body temperature Those suffering from cold, flu, or fever should not perform this Pranayam.
3	Ardha Chandrasana	legs and the core	• tones your thighs, butt, and your arms • stretches your abdominal and back muscles Those suffering from knee pain, frozen shoulder, severe back pain, heart ailments, and high blood pressure should not perform this asana.
4	Ardha Halasana	pelvic region	• strengthens the abdominal muscle • burns fat in the thighs, hips, and abdomen

S. no	Asana	Area it works on	Benefits
			• beneficial for those suffering from diabetes, constipation, indigestion, and weak nerves Those suffering from back pain should not perform this asana.
5	Ardha Matsyendrasana	pancreas, spine, kidneys, stomach, small intestines, liver, and gall bladder	• improves digestion and functioning of the liver • beneficial for kidney patients and diabetics • helps in making the muscles of shoulders and back supple Those suffering from stiff back should perform this asana carefully.
6	Ardha Naukasana	abdomen	• strengthens the abdominal muscles • massages the internal organs • beneficial for diabetic patients Those suffering from hernia, high blood pressure, and heart problems should not perform this asana.
7	Ardha Padma Padottanasana	legs	• improves sense of balance • beneficial for those suffering from constipation, indigestion, and gastroenteritis Those suffering from back pain should not perform this asana.

S. no	Asana	Area it works on	Benefits
8	Pavanmuktasana	back, abdomen, buttocks	• helps cure constipation and releases gas from the stomach. Those suffering from cervical problems should not raise the chin up.
9	Ardha Shalabhasana	lower body, back	• strengthens the lower abdomen, butt, and lower back muscles • cures pain in the thighs and legs Those suffering from lumbar spondylosis should not perform this asana.
10	Ek Pada Ardha Halasana	stomach, thighs	• useful for the lower abdomen and thigh muscles Those suffering from back pain should do this asana carefully.
11	Baddha Padmasana	upper torso, back	• reduces pain from the shoulders, arms, chest, and back muscles Those suffering from arthritis should not perform this asana.
12	Brahma Mudra	neck, spine	• removes stiffness from the neck • beneficial for cervical spondylosis • improves concentration Those suffering from severe cervical spondylosis should perform this asana very carefully.

S. no	Asana	Area it works on	Benefits
13	Bhadrasana	pelvic area, back	• opens groin muscles • straightens the back • beneficial for pregnant women as it helps to ease labour pain People who have very stiff muscles should perform this asana carefully and those suffering from hernia should not perform this asana.
14	Bhastrika Pranayam	all the systems inside the body	• releases toxins from the body • balances the doshas (kapha, pitta, and vata) • supplies more oxygen to the bloodstream Those suffering from heart disease, high blood pressure, and hernia should not perform this Pranayam.
15	Bhramari Pranayam	all the systems inside the body	• beneficial for those suffering from migraine, sinus, and thyroid problems • relaxes the facial muscles and releases tension, making you calm This Pranayam can be performed by anyone.
16	Bhujangasana	spine and abdomen	• improves spinal flexibility • massages the internal organs and digestive tracts Those suffering from heart problems, high blood pressure, and severe back problems should perform this asana carefully.

S. no	Asana	Area it works on	Benefits
17	Chair pose against the wall	thighs	• helps to reduce fat on the thighs You should not do this asana if you have arthritis.
18	Chandranamaskar	spine, legs, arms, abdomen	• helps to relax the mind and body • stretches the spine, hamstrings, and the back of legs • strengthens the legs, arms, back, and stomach muscles
19	Chandrabedhan Pranayam	all the systems inside the body	• cools the system • beneficial for people suffering from high blood pressure, acidity, and stress Those suffering from low blood pressure, and sinus should not do this Pranayam.
20	Chakrasana	abdomen, upper arm, spine	• strengthens the abdominal and calf muscles along with biceps • improves digestion and spinal flexibility Those suffering from high blood pressure and back pain should not perform this asana.
21	Dhanurasana	abdomen, legs, arms, back	• tones arms, legs, stomach, and back muscles Those suffering from heart problems, high blood pressure, and lumbar spondylosis should not perform this asana.

S. no	Asana	Area it works on	Benefits
22	Ek Padasana	limbs, back	• strengthens and tones the arms, legs, and back • improves body and mind balance Beginners and people suffering from severe knee problems should take the support of a wall while doing this asana.
23	Ek Pada Ardha Halasana variation	abdomen, thighs	• useful for your inner as well as outer thigh.
24	Ek Padottanasana	hip, hamstring	• helps to improve the flexibility of the hip and hamstring • strengthens the reproductive system Those suffering from stiff muscles should slowly and gradually get into this posture.
25	Ek Pada Hasta Santolanasana	upper body, legs	• strengthens the arms, chest, abdomen, and legs • creates balance in the body Those suffering from hernia, cervical spondolysis, and frozen shoulders should not perform this asana.
26	Garudasana	upper back, limbs	• tones and strengthens the upper back • improves concentration • strengthens the muscles of the arms, shoulders, and legs Beginners should perform this asana with the support of the wall.

S. no	Asana	Area it works on	Benefits
27	Gomukhasana	back, limbs	• strengthens and tones your arms, legs, and back • relieves back pain, sciatica, and stiffness in the shoulders and neck • beneficial for those suffering from arthritis and dry piles Those suffering from bleeding piles should not perform this asana.
28	Poorna Halasana	back, spine	• stretches the back and the spine • massages the internal organs • beneficial for the digestive and circulatory systems • Remember to do its counterpose Kati Chakrasana, for 15 seconds on each side. Those suffering from cervical spondolysis and stiffness in the spine and shoulders should not perform this asana.
29	Hanumanasana	back, legs	• improves flexibility of the hamstrings, calves, back and shoulder muscles Those suffering from stiff muscles, frozen shoulders, and back pain should not perform this asana.
30	Jalandhara Bandha	all the systems inside the body	• stimulates the secretion in the thyroid gland to balance the hormones in the body Those suffering from cervical spondylosis should not perform this Bandha and people suffering from hypothyroid should check with their doctors before doing it.

S. no	Asana	Area it works on	Benefits
31	Janu Shirshasana	pelvic region, abdomen	• massages the abdominal and pelvic region • reduces fat from the abdomen • increases flexibility of the back Those suffering from slip disc, hernia, and sciatica should not perform this asana.
32	Kapalbhati kriya	all the systems inside the body	• balances and strengthens the nervous system • tones your digestive organs • cleanses the lungs and is good for any respiratory problems Heart patients or people with high blood pressure should avoid this kriya.
33	Konasana	back	• makes the spine flexible • beneficial for people with back and hip pain Those suffering from cervical, lumbar spondylosis and hypertension should not perform this asana.
34	Ardha Kapotasana	abdomen, back	• stretches the hip, abdomen, arms and the back muscles People suffering from arthritis and back pain should not perform this asana.
35	Jalneti kriya	nasal passage	• opens up the blockages in the nose and in the blood vessels on the face • facilitates better flow of blood and oxygen to the facial muscles

S. no	Asana	Area it works on	Benefits
36	Shankhaprakshalana	the entire body	• cleanses the intestinal tract Should be performed only under supervision
37	Sutraneti kriya	nasal passage	• cleanses and clears the nasal blockages Should be performed only under supervision
38	Makarasana	back, abdomen	• relaxes the back muscles and improves digestion Pregnant women should not perform this asana.
39	Marjariasana	neck, back	• improves flexibility in the shoulders, neck, and spine • beneficial for pregnant women but should be performed very carefully without any pressure on the abdomen When performing this asana do not bend the elbows.
40	Matsyasana	neck, abdomen, pelvic area	• makes the nervous system, kidneys, stomach, intestines, and the pelvic organs strong
41	Merudandasana	entire body	• strengthens the abdominal, back, arms, and leg muscles • beneficial for diabetes and any abdominal problems Those suffering from high blood pressure, heart problems, and back pain should not perform this asana.

S. no	Asana	Area it works on	Benefits
42	Naukasana	middle of the body	• tones and strengthens the abdominal muscles • useful for diabeties • helps to create a sense of balance Those suffering from hypertension, heart problems, and lumbar spondylosis should not perform this asana.
43	Natrajasana	back, arms, hips	• strengthens the back, shoulders, arms, and hips • helps to improve concentration Those who suffer from high blood pressure and back problems should not perform this asana.
44	Niralambasana	neck	• reduces cervical pain • relaxes the neck muscles This asana can be done by everybody.
45	Paschimottanasana	abdomen	• tones and massages the abdomen and pelvic region • helps to lose weight in the abdominal region • stretches the back, hamstring muscles, increases flexibility in the hip Those suffering from sciatica, hernia, and slip disc should not perform this asana.
46	Padahastasana	abdomen, spine, back, harmstrings	• improves flexibility of the hamstrings and lower back • massages the internal organs • provides increased blood flow to the upper body People suffering from stiff muscles and back pain should perform this asana carefully.

S. no	Asana	Area it works on	Benefits
47	Pada Prasar Paschimottansan	chest, shoulders, thighs	• massages the internal organs • stretches the inner thighs, muscles under and between the shoulder blades and chest Do not try very hard to reach the final position. Perform this asana slowly and gradually.
48	Padmasana	the entire body and mind	• helps in improving concentration Those who cannot do Padmasana can try this asana with one leg folded as in Ardha Padmasana, till slowly and gradually you are able to do Padmasana. Those suffering from arthritis should not perform this asana.
49	Parighasana	pelvic region, side of the body	• stretches the pelvic region and the groin muscles • burns fat from the sides of the hips or what we commonly refer to as 'love handles'
50	Parivritta Janu Shirshasana	hamstrings, hips	• stretches the hamstring, shoulder, and the sides of the body • helps to melt fat from the side of the hips Those suffering from high blood pressure, cervical spondylosis, and heart problems should not perform this asana.

S. no	Asana	Area it works on	Benefits
51	Parvatasana in Padmasana	upper body, arms	• makes the upper back and shoulder flexible • stretches the arms • recommended for asthmatic patients Those suffering from arthritis or any knee problem should not perform this asana
52	Poorna Triyak Naukasana	entire body especially the abdomen	• strengthens and tones the sides of the body and the abdominal muscles Those suffering from severe back pain should not perform this asana.
53	Sarvangasana	upper body, lungs, thyroid glands	• helps control ageing • useful for those suffering from constipation and hernia People suffering from high blood pressure and heart disease should not perform this asana.
54	Santolanasana	arms, shoulders	• strengthens the arms, chest, abdomen and legs, making the muscles strong • creates balance in the body People suffering from hernia, cervical spondylosis, and frozen shoulder should not perform this asana
55	Sarpasana	upper back, spine, abdomen	• beneficial for all abdominal organs • helps to cure backache • improves posture People suffering from hernia and slip disc should not perform this asana.

S. no	Asana	Area it works on	Benefits
56	Shavasana	entire body	• removes fatigue from the body and relaxes all the muscles • regulates blood pressure • beneficial for those suffering from insomnia, cardiac diseases, and hypertension People suffering from major back problems should place a pillow under their knees while doing this asana.
57	Setubandhasana	back, shoulders, thighs	• strengthens the shoulders and thigh muscles • tones the back • helps to relieve pain due to menstrual cramps This asana is recommended for people having a thyroid problem.
58	Shishpadangu-stanasana	head, thighs, hamstrings	• stretches the hamstrings, thighs, and shoulder blades • improves blood flow towards the head • helps to lose weight in the affected areas Those suffering from heart diseases, high blood pressure, and severe back pain should not perform this asana.
59	Sheetali Pranayam	entire body and mind	• provides a cooling effect to the body • helps to reduce mental tension Those suffering from high blood pressure should not do this Pranayam.

S. no	Asana	Area it works on	Benefits
60	Simhasana	face	• improves eyesight • increases blood circulation in the facial muscles
61	Supta Vajrasana	lower body, abdomen	• increases flexibility of the body • improves blood flow to the lower body improves the capacity of the lungs • helps to cure constipation People suffering from arthiritis, sciatica, slip disc, or back pain should not perform this asana.
62	Supta Tadasana	entire body	• increases flexibility of the body • enhances blood flow to the lower body • improves capacity of the lungs • helps to cure constipation People suffering from arthiritis, sciatica, slip disc, or back pain should not perform this asana.
63	Suryabhedan pranayam	entire body	• creates heat in the body by regulating imbalances of vata and kapha • makes you feel energetic • beneficial for people with low blood pressure People suffering from acidity, hypertension, heart problems, hyperthyroid should not do this Pranayam.

S. no	Asana	Area it works on	Benefits
64	Suryanamaskar	entire body, especially the abdomen, legs, arms, knees	• improves the digestive system • stretches the abdominal muscles • helps to lose weight especially from the stomach area • improves blood circulation
65	Sukhasana	entire body and mind	• relaxes the mind and the body People suffering from arthritis should take the support of a wall and then perform this asana.
66	Tadasana	spine, calves, buttocks	• improves height • improves flexibility of the spine • stretches the calves and tones the buttocks
67	Trataka kriya	eyes	• beneficial for eyes • increases concentration
68	Trikonasana	spine, hamstrings	• makes the spine flexible • strengthens the hamstrings • increases blood flow to the upper body People suffering from cervical, lumbar spondylosis and hypertension should not perform this asana.
69	Ardha Triyak Naukasana	abdomen	• strengthens the obliques and abdominal muscles Those suffering from a severe back pain should not perform this asana.

S. no	Asana	Area it works on	Benefits
70	Triyak Bhujangasana	spine	• improves spinal flexibility • massages internal organs and the digestive system
71	Ugrasana	pelvic region, abdomen, back	• relieves tension from the pelvic region • tones the abdominal organs • stimulates blood circulation to these areas • strengthens the lower back Pregnant women and those suffering from hernia should avoid this asana.
72	Ujjayi Pranayam	entire body and mind	• balances the hormones • improves concentration • beneficial for those who suffer from insomnia and high blood pressure • helps to relieve stress and tension You should not do this Pranayam if you are suffering from heart ailments.
73	Ustrasana	upper body, thighs	• improves digestion • removes stiffness from thighs, abdomen, chest, shoulders, arms, and neck muscles • beneficial for asthmatic patients People suffering from stiff muscles, lumbar and cervical spondolysis should perform the asana carefully.
74	Utkatasana	calf muscles and thighs	• strengthens and tones calves and thighs You should not do this asana if you have arthritis.

S. no	Asana	Area it works on	Benefits
75	Uttanasana	joints like hips, knee, ankles	• strengthens the hip and the thighs • makes the knee, ankle, and back stronger If you are suffering from knee problems you should not perform this asana. Pregnant women should practise this asana slowly with support.
76	Ardha Halasana	abdomen	• strengthens the abdominal muscles • beneficial for those suffering from diabetes, constipation, indigestion, and nervous weakness People suffering from back pain should not do this asana.
77	Uttan Mandukasana	abdomen	• improves efficiency of the lungs • enhances blood flow to the chest and abdomen • tones the abdominal and shoulder muscles People having stiff muscles, frozen shoulder, and cervical spondolysis should perform this asana carefully.
78	Vajrasana	lower body, digestive system	• strengthens the thigh and the calf muscles • beneficial for the digestive system Those suffering from arthritis, severe back pain, and piles should not perform this asana.

S. no	Asana	Area it works on	Benefits
79	Vakrasana	back, abdomen	• beneficial for those suffering from constipation, weak liver, kidney, and stomach diseases • reduces stiffness in the back
80	Vaman Kriya	respiratory system	• helps remove the excess mucous, thereby improving the respiratory functions • helps to remove blocked emotions and unwanted inner and outer conflicts that take place in our lives on a regular basis This kriya has to be practised under the supervision of a yoga expert.
81	Vipreetkarni	head	• directs and enhances the blood flow towards the head • regular practice of this asana keeps your heart, brain, and facial muscles young Those suffering from heart diseases and high blood pressure should not perform this asana.
82	Vrikshasana	lower body	• strengthens the thighs and calf muscles • improves mind and body coordination Beginners should practise this with support.
83	Yoga Mudra	entire body, digestive system	• massages internal organs • improves the digestive system People suffering from severe headaches and high blood pressure should not do this.

S. no	Asana	Area it works on	Benefits
84	Jumping Jack	cardiac system	• improves blood circulation • increases the heart rate People suffering with arthritis, back pain, high blood pressure, and heart patients should avoid this.
85	Sideways Naukasana	oblique muscles	• strength the oblique muscles • tones the abdominal area People suffering from back pain should avoid this asana.
86	Setubandhasana variation (with legs straight)	entire body	• Stretches the entire body like the legs, back, and the abdominal muscles • extremely beneficial for people with drooping and rounded shoulders People with frozen shoulders and back pain should not perform this asana.
87	Dwi Pada Uttan Paschimottanasana	arms, legs	• improves the flexibility of the legs • strengthens the arms • improves concentration. People suffering from back pain and stiff muscles should not perform this asana.
88	Ek Pada Uttan Paschimottanasana	arms, legs, back	• strengthens the leg and arm muscles People suffering from back pain should perform this asana carefully.

S. no	Asana	Area it works on	Benefits
89	Tolangulasana	core of your body	• strengthens the biceps, abdomen, and back muscles • improves digestion • beneficial for people suffering from diabetes and piles People suffering from back pain or slip disc should not perform this asana.
90	Saral Santolanasana	sides of the body, arms	• strengthens the upper body • reduces fat from the outer thighs People suffering from frozen shoulders and cervical spondolysis should not perform this asana.
91	Utkatasana (chair pose) level 1	thighs, butt	• Strengthens the quadriceps • reduces fat from the lower body People suffering from arthritis and varicose veins should not perform this asana.
92	Utkatasana (chair pose) level 3	thighs, butt, calves	• strengthens the quadriceps and calf muscles reduces fat from the lower body People suffering from arthritis, having an injured knee, and varicose veins should not perform this asana.
93	Ek Pada Uttan Angusthasana	legs, back	• increases flexibility in the lower body • improves coordination between the body and the mind People suffering from knee and back pain should do this with utmost care. Beginners should perform it the support of the wall.

S. no	Asana	Area it works on	Benefits
94	Sharnagat Mudra	back	• relaxes the arms, shoulders, neck, back, and abdominal muscles • improves digestion This asana can be done by everybody as it is a relaxing posture.
95	Kati Chakrasana crocodile series	back	• beneficial for people suffering from sciatica and back pain Those suffering from a severe back disease should perform this asana carefully.
96	Ek Pada Vyaghrasana	legs, back	• improves flexibility of the arms • strengthens the leg muscles People suffering from severe back pain should avoid this asana.
97	Ek Pada Ugrasana	legs, back	• relieves tension from the pelvic region • stretches the calf muscles • aligns the back • stimulates blood circulation to the pelvic region, calf and back
98	Chandranamaskar	entire body	• promotes blood circulation • stretches the spine, hamstrings, legs, and strengthens them

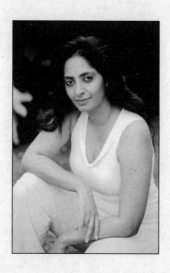

Payal Gidwani Tiwari is one of the most famous fitness and yoga experts of Bollywood. Her clients include Kareena Kapoor, Saif Ali Khan, Rani Mukerji, Sridevi Kapoor, Jacqueline Fernandez, Farah Khan, Tusshar Kapoor, Amrita Arora Ladak, Priya Dutt, Suzanne Roshan, Maria Goretti, Tulip Joshi, Zoa Morani, to name just a few. Payal also conducts yoga workshops for corporates, and runs her wellness brand called Cosmic Fusion (www.cosmicfusion.in), which emphasizes daily fitness and a holistic lifestyle.

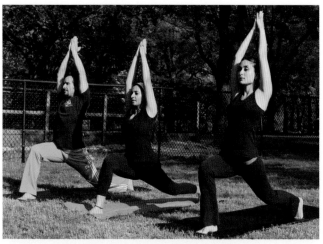

Doing Ardha Chandrasana with Saif and
Kareena at Central Park, New York

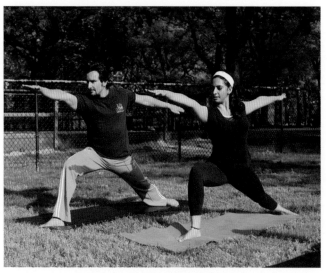

Saif and me doing Virabhadrasana

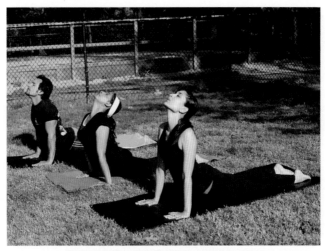

Saif, Kareena and me doing Sarpasana

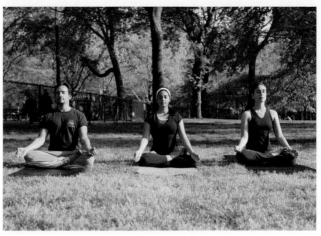

In Padmasana

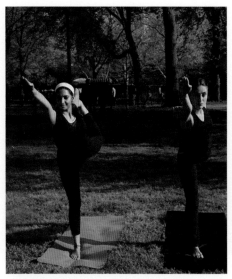

Kareena and me doing Natrajasana

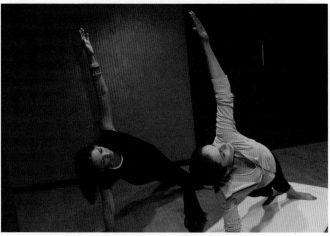

Doing Santolanasana variation 2 with Rani
during the preparation for *Dil Bole Hadippa*

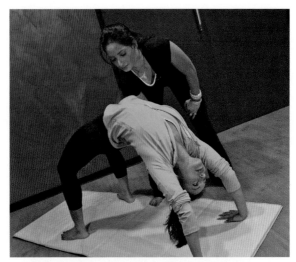

Making Rani do Chakrasana

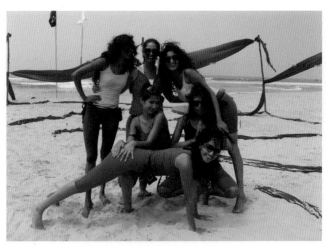

With the models I trained during the
Kingfisher Calendar Hunt 2009

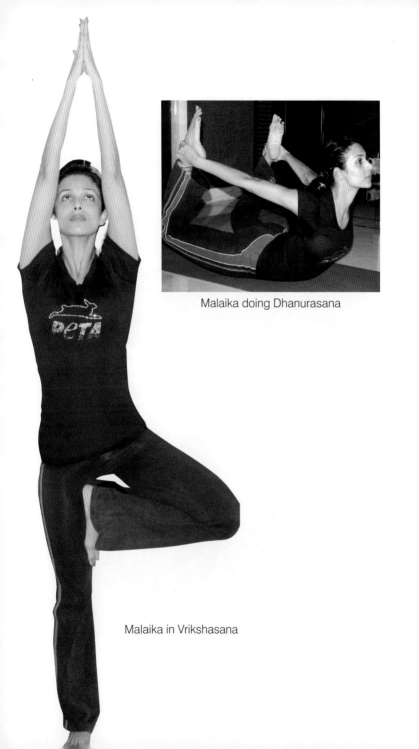

Malaika doing Dhanurasana

Malaika in Vrikshasana

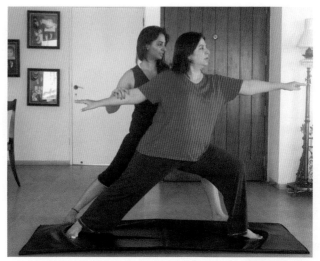

Helping Farah do Virabhadrasana at her residence

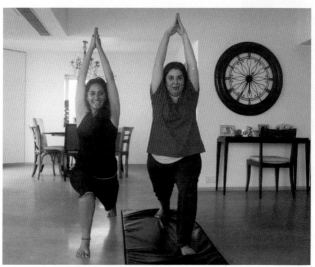

Farah and me in Ardha Chandrasana

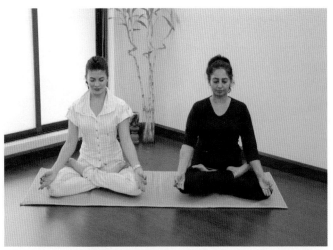

Doing Padmasana with Jacqueline Fernandez at
my studio Cosmic Fusion

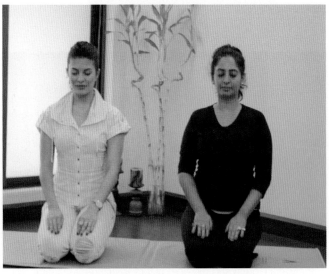

Jacqueline and me in Vajrasana

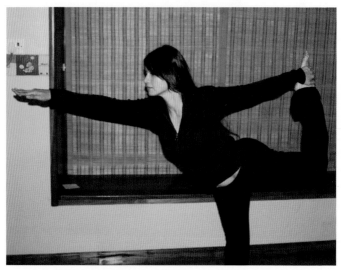

Maria Goretti doing Natrajasana at her home

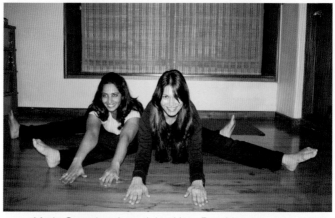

Maria Goretti and me doing Ugra Paschimottanasana

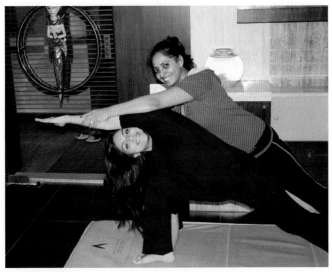

Making Zoa Morani do Konasana variation at
Cosmic Fusion Studio

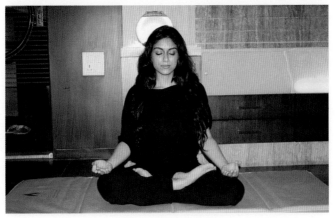

Zoa in Padmasana

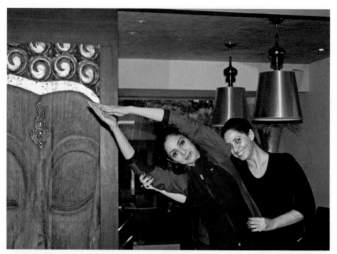

Sridevi getting into side bending Chakrasana at her home

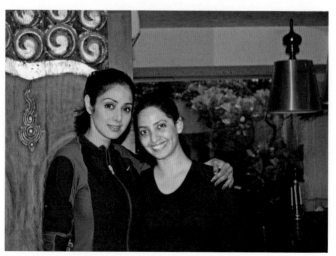

Relaxing with Sridevi after the workout

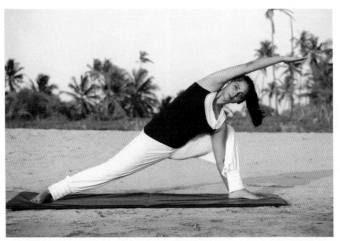

Konasana variation

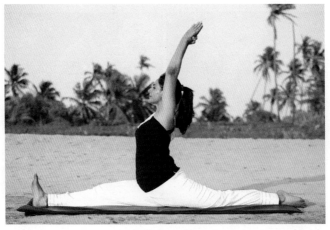

Hanumanasana

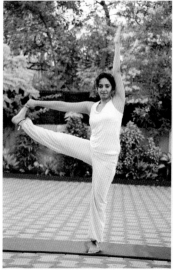

Sideways Ek Pada Uttan
Angusthasana

Natrajasana

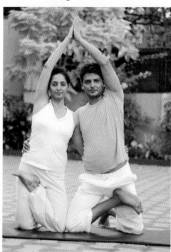

Samtulasana

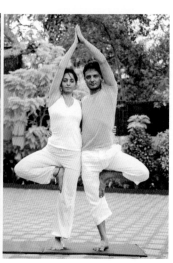

Vrikshasana

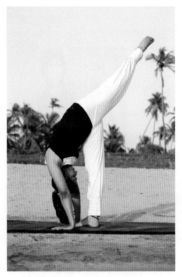

Ek Pada Shirshasana

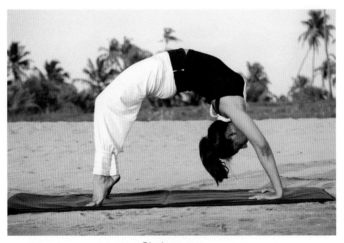

Chakrasana

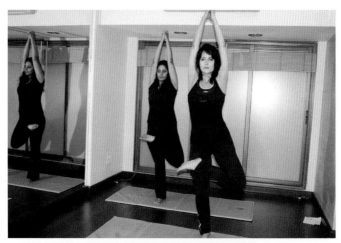

In Ardha Baddha Padmottanasana with Tulip Joshi
at Cosmic Fusion

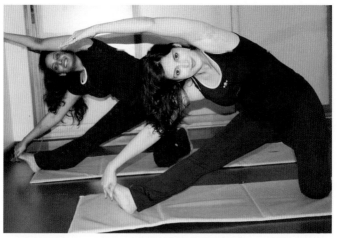

Doing Parighasana with Tulip

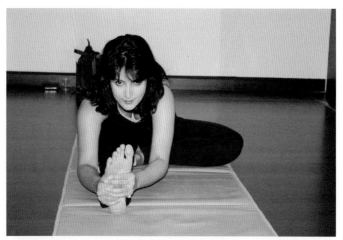

Tulip in Janu Shirshasana

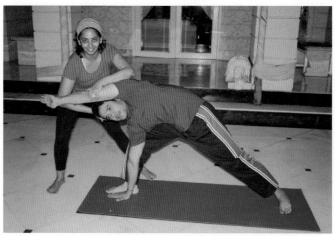

Helping Tusshar Kapoor do Konasana at his home

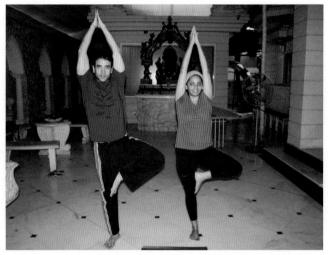

Doing Vrikshasana with Tusshar Kapoor

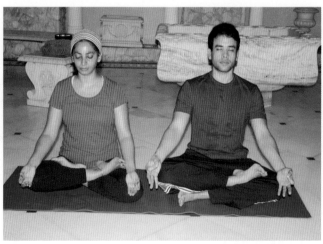

Tusshar Kapoor and me in Gyan Mudra to relax after the workout